"A LITTLE ANXIETY BRINGS OUT THE BEST IN US."

"A life without emotions, anxiety included, would be very drab. Yet too much is debilitating...Excessive anxiety inhibits and defeats us. We have all been frozen by fear or have been unable to perform simple functions in front of an audience that made us nervous.

"...In the chapters to follow we will present a number of specific ways to keep anxiety in check so that it enhances rather than inhibits performance. Anxiety is a fact of existence. It is best to make it work for us rather than against us. There is an old military saying, 'Don't sweat the little stuff.' One might add, 'Everything is little stuff, and if you can't fight or flee, flow.'"

Learn to R...

Learn to Relax

PROVEN TECHNIQUES FOR REDUCING STRESS, TENSION AND ANXIETY FOR PEAK PERFORMANCE

C. EUGENE WALKER, Ph.D

B

BERKLEY BOOKS, NEW YORK

This Berkley book contains the revised text of the original edition. It
has been completely reset in a typeface designed for easy reading and
was printed from new film.

LEARN TO RELAX

A Berkley Book / published by arrangement with
the author

PRINTING HISTORY
Prentice-Hall Inc. edition published 1975
Berkley revised edition / July 1991

ISBN: 0-425-12776-1

A BERKLEY BOOK® TM 757,375
Berkley Books are published by The Berkley Publishing Group,
200 Madison Avenue, New York, New York 10016.
The name "Berkley" and the "B" logo
are trademarks belonging to Berkley Publishing Corporation.

PRINTED IN THE UNITED STATES OF AMERICA

10 9 8 7 6 5 4

To Rita, my sister,
who taught me much about the art of living.

Contents

★

Preface

★

THE first edition of this book proved to be helpful to thousands of people. Hence, after over fifteen years it seemed time to revise and update the contents.

A basic fact of life is that we all experience tension and anxiety as a part of our existence. Sometimes the experience is mild and passes quickly. Sometimes it is agonizingly severe and may last for long periods of time. Although humans have always experienced anxiety, some think that the nature of our civilization and technology may be causing our tensions and anxieties to escalate at a rate faster than our ability to cope with them. It is impossible to know whether this is true. The basic fact of anxiety as a part of living, however, remains with us. Psychologists have developed numerous ways to treat anxiety in those who come for help. In this book you will find these techniques, many of them quite new, explained in such a way that you can use them yourself. These techniques have helped millions of people. It is my hope that they will be useful to you.

One final note: To avoid sexist language and yet not encumber the reader with awkward sentence structure, I have chosen to alternate male and female pronouns from chapter to chapter. I trust that this will not distract the reader from the message of the book.

Learn to Relax

1

What Is Anxiety?

BECAUSE anxiety is such a simple word and such a common experience for all people, it may come as a surprise that psychologists do not really know exactly what it is. In fact, some psychologists have argued that the term itself is so vague and so general that it is useless for precise communication. While this may seem like nonsense—psychology is sometimes called the science of making common sense unintelligible—there are problems in clearly defining what we mean by *anxiety*. The reason is that anxiety is a word that we use to cover a large number of situations. For example, you may say to us that you are anxious. This may be a *subjective feeling* that you are reporting. We may or may not have guessed that you are feeling that way, depending on your outward behavior. If we ask further, we may find that your mind seems to be racing and is full of worries, fears, and ideas that keep recurring. There may be various physical sensations also, but they may not seem to be especially prominent. The anxiety seems to be centered in the head.

Another situation that we would label anxiety is *mental blocking*. For example, if you are very tense about an exam, you may study diligently and know the material thoroughly before the test. When the test is presented, however, sometimes you find to your consternation that your mind is blank;

nothing that was studied can be remembered. Generally, as soon as the exam hour is over, the memory magically returns. Some understanding instructors will allow the student to complete the exam, even though the time is up. Another way of handling this situation is for you to quit trying for a while. You might get a drink of water, take a short walk, sharpen a pencil, or do something of that sort. Often a person in such a situation is trying too hard. Breaking the mental set lets you get a fresh start and get over the blocking.

But you might say that your mind or head is clear, but you are experiencing *physical sensations* or problems that you call anxiety. These may include one or more of the following, as well as a host of others: muscular tightness, nausea, stiff neck, general or localized body pain, respiratory problems, rapid or irregular heartbeat, dry mouth, hot flashes, chills, sweating (especially on the hands), excessive urination, diarrhea, loss of appetite, and sleep disturbances.

On the other hand, you might deny subjective feelings of anxiety, have no mental blocking, and also claim that none of the physical symptoms mentioned above are present. Yet we might insist that you are anxious if we note such *behaviors* as changes in normal speech patterns, stuttering, stammering, distinctive facial expressions, tics or twitches, physical awkwardness, making mental errors, or having accidents. When I was a graduate student of psychology at Purdue University, my peers and I lived under a great deal of tension and anxiety about our studies and our futures. All graduate students feel such pressure. A standing joke with us was to walk up to a fellow student and ask if he was anxious. The correct response to this question was to give a startled response, purse the lips, and say, "Nope."

If you have one or any combination of the signs above, one might say you are anxious, or others might consider you to be anxious. In addition, at different times in one's life or in response to different situations, a person might show different patterns of these signs. We would label them all anxiety. To further complicate matters, studies of all these components indicate that different people experience different patterns and combinations of the above in the *same* situation. They would all say, however, that they were *anxious*. So the word does cover a multitude of experiences— some of which are subjective feelings, some mental reactions, some physical reactions, and some of which are changes in behavior. Anxiety seems to be everywhere and in everyone.

Excessive anxiety is considered to be one of the major symptoms of neurosis, and some have speculated that the nature of humans may be to be neurotic, at least in civilized society as we know it today. Some ethologists and anthropologists argue that this is the case because in our evolutionary history, the survival of the "beast" known as Homo sapiens depended on a combination of physical aggressiveness and mental foresight. This "beast," however, now finds itself in a society that permits powers of foresight to run wild (even feeds and exaggerates them with communications media) but forbids the use of physical force or aggression as a solution to problems. The famous physiologist, Walter B. Cannon, demonstrated that the nervous system of humans prepares them physically for fight or flight in the face of danger. Unfortunately, in our complex civilization, neither of these is very effective. If we are physically aggressive, we are likely to be arrested. If we attempt to flee our obligations, we will be detected and returned to the situation. Thus, Homo sapiens may be like cornered animals that experience a chronic state of anxiety (or neurosis) in our complex world. In the later chapters of this book, we will see that such a pessimistic prospect is not inevitable.

Because anxiety is such a vague term, it might be helpful to define several related terms that describe human experience in this area. Psychologists differ in their use of these terms depending on their ideas about personality and psychotherapy. The following definitions are simple ones that will do for our discussion.

While there is no completely adequate definition of **anxiety**, we might refer to it as the reaction we have to a situation where we believe our well-being is endangered or threatened in some way. This may be any form of well-being. We may feel that our physical safety is in danger, or our success in our job, or our self-esteem, or the well-being of someone important to us, as in the case of the parent anxiously waiting for a child to return from a date. To say you are "nervous" is pretty much synonymous with saying you are "anxious." **Tension** may be thought of as chronic, usually low-level anxiety that is experienced as a part of an ongoing situation in which we are involved.

Fear is intense anxiety experienced in response to a specific threat. A **phobia** is an intense, incapacitating and irrational fear attached to a specific thing or situation. Most people have some phobias, whether they are of blood, bugs, snakes, airplanes, or whatever. We used to give fancy Greek names to each phobia, claustrophobia (fear of enclosed places), acrophobia (fear of high places), hydrophobia (fear of water), and so forth. But clinicians now just label the problem as a phobia and state plainly what the object is. In chapter two we present a technique that eliminates phobias in a relatively short period of time.

Unconscious anxiety may mean many things, but basically, as we might expect, it is anxiety of which we are not consciously aware. For example, often we don't realize how tense or anxious we were about a matter until it has passed. The relief we feel at that moment makes us reflect on the past and decide that we were anxious at the time. Yet, we did not consciously label it as such at the time it was occurring.

Free-floating anxiety describes a situation where intense anxiety seems unexpectedly to attack a person, only to go away and return later. Generally you realize that you are under a great deal of general tension or strain but are unable to connect specific events with the attacks.

Panic is a condition in which the anxiety has become so great that the person loses control of the situation. The person often becomes confused and may do bizarre things. It is a very painful and unpleasant experience. Many emotionally disturbed people seem to live in a chronic state of panic or near panic. When we deal with them, it helps if we keep this in mind. Gentleness, patience, and help in structuring things so they can handle them can go a long way with such people.

Stress is a term that has come to be used almost synonymously with anxiety, but it includes an extra and important dimension. In physical sciences, stress refers to the effect of placing a load on an object such as weight on a bridge. Obviously the bridge can hold only so much weight before it breaks. Other factors such as wind and temperature may also impinge on the bridge's ability to hold. In psychology we use the term stress to describe the amount of pressure from the environment that you can handle before you begin to develop problems in coping. Thus, Richard Lazarus, one of the foremost authorities on stress, offers the following definition: "Psychological stress is a particular relationship between the person and the environment that is appraised by the person as taxing or exceeding his or her resources and endangering his or her well-being." (Richard

S. Lazarus and Susan Folkman, *Stress, Appraisal, and Coping*. New York: Springer Publishing Co., 1984, p. 19). This definition emphasizes the interaction between the "load" from the environment and the resiliency of the person.

One of the pioneers in the area of stress research was Hans Selye. Selye identified three stages of reaction to a stressor. The first is alarm and mobilization in which the body begins to battle the stressor. The second is resistance in which the body attempts to withstand the pressure. This is followed by exhaustion and disintegration where the body breaks down and physical symptoms occur such as ulcers, high blood pressure, headaches, infections, and so forth. Selye called this the general adaptation syndrome and felt that it explained the appearance of psychosomatic diseases as well as our sometimes increased susceptibility to organic illness. In extreme or prolonged cases, the result is death.

From what we have said so far, we might get the idea that anxiety is the great enemy of human beings. This is only partly true, however. Anxiety is a lot like pain. We prefer to experience as little of it as possible, but it serves a very useful purpose in alerting us and activating our defenses in times of danger. Moderate amounts of anxiety motivate us to plan for future events and increases our ability to cope with situations as they occur. The increased strength of the person who is afraid or the person who admits he works better under a little pressure are examples of the beneficial nature of anxiety. I recall, when preparing for the major comprehensive examinations that would determine whether I would receive my degree in psychology, that I became much more mentally alert than usual. I found myself able to read faster than usual and developed almost a photographic memory for what I read, which was not the usual case with me. One reason for this was that the exams were given in January, and as one who considers athletics an art form, I could hardly spend much time preparing for the exam until the "repertory season" of football bowl games was completed.

It is when anxiety becomes excessive that it is a problem. Those who have studied human activation have noted that this is a common feature of many motivating forces. When they are moderate, increasing the amount leads to heightened and better performance. Eventually, however, a peak is reached and any additional amount results in deterioration of the performance. This is certainly the case with anxiety. A little brings out the best in us. A life without emotions, anxiety included, would be very drab. Yet, too much is debilitating. This is part of the fascination of amusement parks. We can administer small amounts of anxiety to ourselves in controlled conditions and feel the joy of dissipating it immediately. Likewise, thriller books and movies are fun because they excite and activate us with an exhilarating feeling in a situation that we know is really quite safe. The person who enjoys challenges does the same thing in real life. We would not enjoy amusement parks, however, if our lives were really in great danger on every ride. Nor would we welcome challenges or tasks in our lives that we were not able to cope with. Such situations would be destructive and debilitating rather than pleasurable. Excessive anxiety inhibits and defeats us. We have all been frozen by fear or have been unable to perform simple functions in front of an audience that made us nervous.

I recall another amazing revelation of this effect of anxiety from my undergraduate days in college. I was taking a course in French, and each day we were assigned translations to do at night that we were to recite the next day in class. I used to labor over these translations for hours each night, looking up every word and puzzling over the syntax to make the translation as close to perfect as possible. It was always embarrassing to make a mistake in front of the whole class. One day I failed to get the translation done ahead of time and had decided to cut class. On the way across campus I ran into my French instructor. I explained to him that I had not had time to do the translation for the day and did not want to take his time without being prepared. He suggested that I come along anyway and just listen. When it was my turn to recite, however, he asked if I would like to try it even though I wasn't prepared. I decided I would and found to my surprise that I was able to read the lesson without hesitation as though it were in English. I stopped only at words in the new vocabulary for the day and easily went on after they were supplied by the instructor. The fact is that by removing all pressure to perform and anxiety about being so precise, I was able to do better than ever. I felt no pressure because, after all, I hadn't prepared and couldn't be expected to do very well. I had never been able to do that before and have never been able to do it since. That was the only time I was able to approach a translation completely free of inhibiting anxieties.

In the chapters to follow we will present a number of specific ways to keep anxiety in check so that it enhances rather than inhibits performance. Anxiety is a fact of existence. It is best to learn to make it work for us rather than against us. There is an old military saying, "Don't sweat the little stuff." One might add, "Everything is little stuff, and if you can't fight or flee, flow."

2

Systematic Desensitization

★

MANY of the anxieties that people experience are due to what psychologists call conditioned reactions. Simply stated, what psychologists mean is that things that frequently occur together in our experience become linked or associated with one another so that we respond to them in the same, or a highly similar, way when they happen again. Thus, if we are made anxious or afraid in the presence of certain factors (psychologists refer to them as stimuli), these same factors or stimuli will make us anxious later when they occur, even if the situation in reality no longer poses an actual threat. For example, you may have had a number of experiences as a child in which a person in authority, such as a school principal, police officer, or guard, frightened and perhaps punished you in some way. Your reaction as an adult to someone in authority may produce considerably more anxiety than the situation really calls for. This is because of the previous conditioning of strong anxiety to this type of person. A person so conditioned might be driving along a highway obeying all traffic laws and see a police car pull up behind. She may feel considerable anxiety at the approach of the car. If the police officer stops her, the driver may have many symptoms of anxiety such as a pounding heart, rapid breathing, muscular tenseness, stuttering and stammering speech. Of course, this is an overreaction to the situation. This person was breaking no law, and the officer may only want to tell her that a taillight is broken or warn of a road hazard ahead. At worst, the driver may have broken a minor traffic law, which would cost a fine of a few dollars. For many, however, the situation evokes anxiety near panic. Such effects often result from conditioned reactions.

Many of our emotions seem to be largely based on such responses. Conditioned reactions are somewhat similar to reflexes, but they are learned rather than inherited. Their automatic or ''reflexive'' character, however, explains why it is hard to discuss things rationally with someone who is emotionally involved in a situation. Such a person is responding more through conditioned reactions to the present stimuli than relating to the realities of the situation. It also explains why we can tell ourselves that the next time a situation occurs we are not going to let it upset us and are going to handle it a certain way, only to find that when it does occur, we respond pretty much as we always have. This is the nature of conditioned reactions.

Now, if many of our anxieties are conditioned reactions, what can we do about them? Are we the victims of our traumatic past, or can we overcome such anxieties? Fortunately we can overcome them. In fact, they are amazingly easy to overcome if we work at them in the right way. For decades psychologists have studied conditioned reactions in research laboratories all over the world. A clinical procedure for eliminating conditioned anxiety reactions, developed by Dr. Joseph Wolpe, a psychiatrist, makes use of the basic principles learned from research. It is called systematic desensitization. If done properly, it works almost every time.

Let's use an example to show how you can use systematic desensitization on your own. Suppose authority persons are your problem. The first step would be to sit down with some index cards and on each card write a different situation or enxperience that causes you anxiety in this area. After you have a stack of cards, place them in order, with the one that causes least anxiety on top and the one that causes most anxiety on the bottom. Your list might look something like this (least anxiety-causing at top, most at bottom):

1. Walking past and greeting one of the bosses at work who is only a little older than myself.
2. Walking past and greeting one of the bosses at work who is considerably older than myself—one with gray hair and a gruff but somewhat pleasant demeanor.
3. Encountering one of the bosses who is only a little older than myself in the coffee-break room, where we will have to talk and have coffee together.
4. Encountering one of the bosses who is considerably older than myself—with gray hair and a gruff but somewhat pleasant demeanor—in the coffee-break room, where we will have to talk and have coffee together.
5. Having one of the bosses who is only a little older than myself watch me, without seeming pleased or displeased, while I work.
6. Having one of the bosses who is considerably older than myself—with gray hair and a gruff but somewhat pleasant demeanor—watch me while I work, without seeing pleased or displeased.
7. Having one of the bosses who is only a little older than myself watch me while I work and seeming to be displeased with what I am doing.
8. Having one of the bosses who is considerably older than myself—with gray hair and a gruff but somewhat pleasant demeanor—watch me while I work

and seem to be displeased with what I am doing.

9. Having one of the bosses who is only a little older than myself watch me while I work and make a slightly critical comment to me after watching for a while.

10. Having one of the bosses who is considerably older than myself—with gray hair and a gruff but somewhat pleasant demeanor—watch me while I work and make a slightly critical comment to me after watching for a while.

11. Having one of the bosses who is only a little older than myself watch me while I work and make a very critical comment after watching for a while.

12. Having one of the bosses who is considerably older than myself—with gray hair and a gruff but somewhat pleasant demeanor—watch me while I work and make a very critical comment after watching for a while.

13. Attending a conference in the office of one of the bosses who is only a little older than myself to discuss something about my work that should be improved.

14. Attending a conference in the office of one of the bosses who is considerably older than myself—with gray hair and a gruff but somewhat pleasant demeanor—to discuss something about my work that should be improved.

15. Attending a conference with several bosses both young and old to discuss something about my work that should be improved.

Next, you have to learn to relax completely. Believe it or not, you can actually train yourself to do this rather easily. First sit in a comfortable chair or lie on a couch or bed.

Then say something like the following to yourself: "I am going to relax completely. I will relax my forehead and scalp. I will let all the muscles of my forehead and scalp relax and become completely at rest. All of the wrinkles will smooth out of my forehead and that part of my body will relax completely. Now I will relax the muscles of my face. I will just let them relax and go limp. There will be no tension in my jaw. Next I will relax my neck muscles. Just let them become tranquil and allow all of the pressure to leave them. My neck muscles are relaxing completely. Now I will relax the muscles of my shoulders. That relaxation will spread down my arms to the elbows, down the forearm to my wrist, hands, and fingers. My arms will just dangle from the frame of my body. I will now relax the muscles of my chest. I will let them relax. I will take a deep breath and relax, letting all of the tightness and tenseness leave. My breathing will now be normal and relaxed, and I will relax the muscles of my stomach. Now I will relax all of the muscles up and down both sides of the spine and let that relaxation spread throughout my back. Now I will relax the waist, buttocks, and thighs down to my knees. Now the relaxation will spread to the calves of my legs, ankles, feet, and toes. I will just lie here and continue to let all of my muscles go completely limp. I will become completely relaxed from the top of my head to the tips of my toes."

If you try this one or two times, you will be amazed at just how relaxed you can become. If you have trouble doing this at first, you might try purposely tensing the muscles of various parts of your body a few times and then letting them relax completely immediately following the forced tension. This will teach you to discriminate clearly between the tense and relaxed states and train you in producing relaxation at will. Go through each of the muscle groups mentioned above (forehead and scalp, face, neck, shoulders, etc.) and learn to relax them one by one. You may spend one or two sessions learning to relax some of the muscles that are hard for you to relax. Then go through the whole procedure in one sitting. You will find yourself very relaxed at this point.

After you are completely relaxed, you are ready to begin the systematic desensitization. Take the top card from the pile and look at it. Then close your eyes and visualize the situation described on it as vividly as you can in your imagination. Imagine it occurring and imagine that you are really there. As you do that, you may experience some anxiety. If so, *stop* the imaginary scene *at once* and go back to relaxing. Relax all of the muscles again. In general, taking just a deep breath or two and letting all of the muscles rest will do the job. If, however, you need to, go through the whole relaxation sequence in your mind again, muscle by muscle.

When you are again completely relaxed, wait a few seconds. Then look at the card and imagine the scene once more. If you feel anxiety, make your mind turn blank, stop imagining the scene, and go back to relaxing. Do this over and over until you can imagine the scene without feeling anxiety. It may take only a couple of times, or it may take fifteen to twenty times, but repeat it until you can imagine the scene without feeling anxiety. When you have accomplished this, go on to the second scene. Continue in this manner until you have gone through all the cards.

It is best to work on the scenes like this for about a half hour at a time. You may want to do it every day or every other day or only a couple of times a week, depending on your schedule and how quickly you want to conquer the anxiety. Usually, from one session to the next, it is a good idea to start by going over the last item or two from the previous session that you were able to imagine without anxiety.

A variation of the above procedure, used by some people, is to tape record a vivid description of the scene in advance. They then relax and listen to the tape. If they feel anxious, they shut the tape off and relax. When calm, they rewind the tape and begin again.

When you have completed the above process for one of the scenes on a card, you will find that this situation—the thought of which used to cause stabbing pains of anxiety—can now be thought of calmly, without disturbance. You have been desensitized. To make the treatment complete, you should now calmly go over in your mind what is the right thing to do in that situation. Make plans to actually do the right thing the next time the situation occurs. You will be amazed to find that your previous anxiety kept you so uptight that you avoided thinking or planning in this area; it prevented you from thinking clearly when you were in the situation. This will all be different now. It is a good idea, as you desensitize yourself to the scenes on the cards, to plan how to handle such situations and then seek out several occasions when you can practice doing better. Some people go through the relaxation procedure just before confronting the real situation. Others just take a deep breath and get as relaxed and composed as they can. Many of my patients have been so elated by the effects of this treatment that they have deliberately sought out situations that previously caused them great anxiety, frustration, and failure.

Once you have desensitized yourself to the situations and experienced them a few times in real life, you will find that they are actually conquered and cause you no discomfort at all. It may seem almost too good to be true, but it does work.

If you have trouble going through the procedure alone,

you might want to enlist the help of a friend. Often you can arrange to trade roles and desensitize each other. If you do this, have the friend instruct you step by step to relax all of your muscles and then describe the scene vividly to you while you stay relaxed. You will need to tell the friend enough details about the scene so that she can weave an imaginary story, one you can really put yourself into and experience. If you feel anxiety at any time, signal the friend by raising the index finger of your right hand. The friend should, at that instant, tell you to turn off your imagination, make your mind go blank, and return to relaxing. When you are relaxed, the process can begin again.

Another way of handling conditioned anxiety that in most cases works just as well as the preceding method, and better in some, is called *in vivo* desensitization. The term *in vivo* simply means, in this case, "in real life." To do this you again make a list of situations and arrange them in order as before. This time, however, skip the imagination part and simply plan in advance how to handle each situation. Then seek out the least anxiety-provoking situation, relax, and carry out your plan. Analyze the results after each try and figure out better ways to respond and handle the situation the next time. Then do it again. Repeat this until you conquer one item on the list, then go on to the next and the next until you are comfortable with each and can handle all of them. Remember that "he who would move mountains must start with the pebbles at the foot of the hill."

As an example of real-life desensitization, suppose you have a lot of anxiety in social situations. After thinking about it you might develop a hierarchy that looks like this (least anxiety-causing at top, most at bottom):

1. Making small talk with a stranger at a bus stop.
2. Having a fairly extended conversation with a

stranger in the doctor's waiting room.

3. Meeting a new person for the first time and talking only briefly with her after being introduced by a mutual friend on the street as you happen to run into one another.

4. Meeting a new person at a party and having to make conversation for a few minutes.

5. Meeting several new people at a party and making small talk.

6. Meeting a new person who joins you and some mutual friends for dinner.

7. Meeting several new people who join you and some mutual friends for dinner.

8. Being the only new person at a dinner party who must meet several people for the first time, sit at a table of strangers, and have dinner with them.

The way to attack the above problem would be to take the first item and look for naturally occurring occasions or even arrange for occasions to occur in which you can experience the event. You should prepare for the occasion in a way that is logical and appropriate. Being prepared is half the battle. In the above example, you might make it a point to read the newspaper to glean some topics to talk about. You might go over in your mind various pleasantries that seem to contribute to a congenial encounter. You might have an appropriate joke or anecdote in the back of your mind. You might search the other person's interests, once you meet, for one you share. A compliment on how one looks or on something the person said will seldom lead you astray and will often make a friend for life. The point is, plan in advance how you will handle the occasion. Then when you are in the situation, work out what you have planned. As a boy, I used to work on a truck farm. The foreman had a large sign on the blackboard at the barn that read, "Plan the work and work the plan." It's good advice.

Just before you enter the situation, go through the relaxation procedure or at least take a few deep breaths, shrug your shoulders, and get completely relaxed. Then go in and do the best you can.

After it is over, think about and analyze how things went. Learn from each experience how to perform better next time. Then do it again. Eventually the anxiety will be gone and you will have developed a repertoire of skills to handle such situations. At that point, you will no longer need the elaborate plans. It will just come naturally.

Be sure to start with the least anxiety-provoking situation. Go on to the next highest and the next only after the ones below it have been conquered. Success depends on a careful, systematic attack.

Looking at the example above, you can see that it deals with social situations involving strangers. Obviously you could make up similar hierarchies involving friends or involving different types of socialization (for example, job interviews or public speaking) or a variety of other things. Most people have been conditioned to react with anxiety to enough situations that they may make up several hierarchies dealing with different areas and work through them. If you have more than one hierarchy at a time that you want to work on, you can work a little on each in every session or go through one completely in a series of sessions and then begin the next.

Some people have used an approach that is in between the imagination approach and the real-life approach discussed above. It is called behavioral rehearsal. In this, you rehearse things with a friend that you would like to do without anxiety. For example, in a job interview, have a friend play the part of the interviewer. The friend can play the part of different kinds of interviewers (stern, hostile, friendly, and so on), and you can practice being calm and responding to the questions. At the end, you can discuss how you might have better handled the situation. Then try it again. Do it over and over until you act without anxiety. The different types of interviews and different types of interviewers can be arranged in hierarchies and worked on using this method.

The hardest part of using these procedures is developing the hierarchies. Often just what it is that makes us anxious seems vague, hard to define or separate out from other factors. The basic strategy is to keep the scenes as simple and straightforward as possible. The best way to start is simply to write down on cards as many situations that involve anxiety as possible without worrying about categories or hierarchies. After you have done that, sort them out into logical categories involving one dimension or a couple of dimensions that seem to go together well. Each of these piles will become a hierarchy of its own. Read over all the items in a given pile and fill in the gaps by writing new cards that obviously would fit in with the ones already written. Extend the range upward and downward by making up more- or less-extreme situations. Eventually you will develop a hierarchy with ten to twenty-five items. If you have too many more than that, break it into two or more hierarchies.

Many times people also wonder if they are including the "right" things in their hierarchies. The best way to handle this is to make them as specific and as close to real life as you can. If they are specific real-life situations that make you anxious, they are right for the hierarchy.

When you start the desensitization procedure, if you have trouble staying relaxed and getting past the first item on the hierarchy, you have started out with one that is too threatening. Write some less anxiety-provoking items, and extend your list downward. If you reach a point at which you have conquered an item but the next one on the list does not seem to be getting any better, say, after fifteen or twenty trials, you probably have made too big a jump. Write some additional items that would logically fit in between the two, and work on them.

Sometimes we have anxiety about an event that doesn't seem to have a logical hierarchy to go with it. Often this is a very unique event, sometimes one that will happen only once in our lives. For example, your upcoming wedding might be causing anxiety. The way to use the systematic desensitization procedure for such events is to imagine the whole event step by step, from beginning to end while staying relaxed. At the first sign of anxiety, stop, make your mind turn blank, then go back to the beginning and start over. Keep this up until you can imagine the whole thing without anxiety. You will find yourself much more relaxed when the event actually occurs than if you had not done this.

One further tip: Imagination, behavioral rehearsal, and in vivo desensitization all work on essentially the same principle. We generally use the imagination and rehearsal procedures for situations that don't occur often enough in real life to make the in vivo system practical or when the situation is so anxiety provoking that we are too terrified to try it in real life. In vivo desensitization should be used as often as possible alone or following the other two methods.

The procedures presented in this chapter work well and can be applied to a large number of anxieties in various areas of life. Since they are based on research findings, they must be done correctly to work. Some people have trouble knowing how to get started or run into difficulties along the way. If this happens, it is best to consult a professional psychologist for assistance. Often the psychologist will be able to give you some advice on how to handle the problems you are having so that you can continue on your own. Sometimes the psychologist may feel that your situation is sufficiently difficult that it would be best for you to see her regularly for a period of time to work on the problems under supervision. This is particularly true if you have major panic attacks or suffer from more serious problems such as agoraphobia (fear of leaving one's home or appearing in public). These problems are beyond the scope of the present book but have been intensively studied in recent years. They can be treated readily by medication and professional psychotherapy. To locate a suitable therapist, call the chair of the psychology or psychiatry department at a nearby university and ask for the names of psychologists or psychiatrists in your area who practice behavior therapy using systematic desensitization.

3

Relaxation Exercises

★

EVERYONE who has gazed at the product of a bodybuilding program or who has watched a skilled athlete perform has been impressed with what can be done to develop and train the muscles of the body through regular, diligent practice. Recent developments in the field of psychology indicate that considerable conscious control can also be exerted over basic physiological processes that were previously thought to be more or less automatic and not subject to such intentional control. Patients have been taught to control heart rate, blood pressure, body temperature, brain waves, and other functions through training. The technique is generally referred to as biofeedback. The basic strategy is to arrange for the individual to receive some type of recognizable feedback when the body process is going in the desired direction and a different type of feedback when it isn't. For example, if you were trying to relax, you might have an apparatus attached that would monitor muscle tension and indicate by a sound what the muscle was doing. Typically the muscle on the forehead is used because it is easy to connect to the electrodes and provides a fairly good index of overall muscle tension. If tension in the muscle begins to increase, the sound becomes louder and faster. As the muscle relaxes, the sound becomes softer and slower. By giving the person this kind of feedback, it is rather easy to train a person to relax. This, of course, is very worthwhile. Use of biofeed-back techniques, however, requires expensive equipment and highly trained personnel to operate it.

Yet it is possible to train yourself to relax your muscles without either. You can learn to do it easily on your own. If relaxation procedures are practiced with regularity, the level of tension and anxiety can be reduced significantly. These procedures may be thought of as relaxation *exercises*. Just as physical exercise trains and strengthens the muscles, making it possible for us to accomplish physical activities that we could not do otherwise, relaxation exercises increase our ability to tolerate stress and to remain calm in the face of life's pressures and problems. This is a crude analogy, of course, but it is helpful to think about it in these terms. The nervous system does not increase in size or change in the same way muscles do with exercise. But with a program of relaxation exercises, the nervous system's functional capacity does change in a very similar way.

Many anxious people feel fairly well in the morning but find themselves becoming more and more tense as the day wears on. By the end of the day they are so tied in knots that they can't enjoy their evening meal. They later find themselves sitting in agony in front of the TV with heartburn, muscular tightness, nausea, a splitting headache, and a general feeling of pain and discomfort. They are unable to relax. What causes this is that during the day minor threats and problems generate tension and anxiety. This makes them uncomfortable and makes them worry about the fact that they are not feeling well and whether there will be more threats and problems as the day wears on and . . . tomorrow. They begin to wonder if they will be able to cope with them indefinitely. Thus, problems, tension, and worry develop into a closed-loop system that maintains itself rather than being dissipated. The net result is a spiral effect, with anxiety increasing at a steady pace, until it is almost unbearable by the end of the day. To stop this process it is necessary to interrupt the feedback, thus breaking the spiral.

One of the simplest ways to accomplish this is to use the relaxation procedure discussed in chapter two. Do it as an exercise, just the way you would do a physical exercise if you wanted to get in top physical shape. You should do it three or four times a day, every day. Once at midmorning, once at noon, once in the evening, and once at bedtime are the best occasions. Go through the process of relaxing all the muscles, and then stay relaxed for three to five minutes. After that, you can get up and go about your business. You will find that you are much more relaxed and calm following the exercise. It should take you only five minutes each time or a total of fifteen to twenty minutes per day. The payoff in reduced anxiety leading to a happier and longer life is well worth the effort.

Some people find it difficult to find time to do the exercise. If you work at a job where you get coffee breaks, that is a good time. You will still have time for your coffee afterward. Of course, too much coffee can make you tense, so you might want to use the entire time for relaxation and skip the cup of coffee. If you don't have coffee breaks, you can go to the rest room at an appropriate time and go through the procedure there. All jobs have a provision for going to the rest room. Also, if you work in a busy place, the rest room is the best place to do the exercise. Usually it is quieter there, and more privacy is afforded.

Again, the procedure interrupts the feedback loop that is causing the anxiety to spiral. The spiral effect ceases, allowing the anxiety to dissipate. Instead of steadily increasing anxiety until you are in misery by the end of the day, you return periodically to a calm, resting state and start over.

At the end of the day you are much more relaxed and less fatigued.

The above exercise can also be used before some type of recreational activity. For example, you can sit down and go through the exercise just before reading a book or watching a TV program. You will then find yourself very relaxed and more able to enjoy the recreation.

Another useful variation is to perform the exercise and then allow yourself to drift off into a nap. You will awaken very relaxed and refreshed. This also is an excellent technique to combat insomnia. To use it for insomnia, get in bed and go through the procedure as indicated. After you are fully relaxed, slowly think the word *sleep* over and over in your mind. Generally, I teach this to a patient in my office. The next time the patient returns for an appointment, I ask how it went. The answer is usually, "It worked very well. In fact, after the first time or two, I never got to the end. I fell asleep in the middle."

Once you have learned to relax using the procedure above, you will often be able to get into the completely relaxed state in a matter of seconds, without going through each set of muscles from head to toe. You will need only to sit or lie in a comfortable position, take a deep breath, exhale, and let all your muscles go limp. The relaxation will be almost instantaneous. This is obviously an ability worth cultivating. It does take diligent systematic effort, however, just as does developing a muscular physique. For those who have trouble learning to relax, it is possible to see a professional therapist who can help by using biofeedback. Such training is often well worth the time and expense.

Some people like to make these relaxation exercises more interesting by using techniques of meditation along with the relaxation. There are numerous approaches to meditation, most of which derive from Oriental philosophy and religion.

Scientific research with these techniques has indicated that they do in fact affect bodily and mental processes in beneficial ways when practiced correctly. People who practice them are often able to achieve a considerable degree of bodily relaxation and mental calmness. They also report that meditation is emotionally a very rewarding experience leading to deeper insight into themselves and their surroundings.

If you want to try these techniques, you must first get in the right position. The lotus position is the most common one. Sit on the floor and cross your legs so that your right foot rests on your left thigh and your left foot rests on your right thigh. Next, make your back into a straight column, resting on the base of your legs and buttocks, so that it is comfortable and requires no strain to keep the back straight. If you put a pillow under your buttocks, this usually will give you a firm, comfortable base. Keep your head and neck comfortably erect. Rest your hands in your lap. The eyes may be kept open and focused at a point a few feet in front of the body, or they may be closed.

This position is, of course, rather difficult for many people to assume. If you have that problem, get as close to it as you comfortably can and then *gently* stretch the muscles each time you do the exercise. Eventually you will be able to do it.

An alternative is generally referred to as the tailor position. For this one, sit with your buttocks on a cushion and fold the legs in front of you so that the right foot is under the left knee and the left foot is under the right knee. Still another possibility is to sit in a straight-backed chair, with your feet firmly on the floor, back and head erect, arms in the lap. Choose the one that best fits your anatomy and physical condition. It is important that you be comfortable.

Once in position, sway back and forth awhile to get completely comfortable. Then take a few deep breaths. With each breath, let go a little and allow your muscles to relax. Mentally you should begin to clear your mind of the business and rushing that characterizes our lives. Begin to adopt a passive, detached attitude of observation. Do not try to achieve a certain state or guide your thinking. Just let the attitude grow.

Having done this, you are ready for specific meditation exercises. One Taoist exercise directs the person to concentrate attention on the center of the torso at about the level of the navel. Thoughts, as they arise, should be "placed" at this level of the body and consciousness should be shifted to the solar plexus (an area in "the pit of the stomach" where numerous nerves and blood vessels meet). Thoughts take on a different meaning, and one develops a different awareness when things are experienced in this manner. This particular exercise has been the occasion for considerable ridicule about people who sit and contemplate their navels, but if practiced correctly it is a stimulating experience for many.

Another exercise is to concentrate on the feelings and sensations of the existence as a being. Or you can observe the process of your mind at work in thought. Watch your thoughts develop, feel them, and see how they are formed. Sometimes you may want to take an object and see it as an existence equivalent to yourself. You may want to meditate on a particular person, physically present with you or not. You may sometimes want to take a significant object from your past with pleasant connotations and meditate on it— such things as an old photograph, a school paper, a flower from your scrapbook, or some similar object.

Some people find it very pleasant to take a fantasy trip while meditating. If you want to do this, think about a place you have been that you liked a great deal. Reexperience it. Transport yourself mentally to the spot. See what is going on. You can concentrate on seeing it exactly as it was when you were there or on how you think it would be now. You can concentrate on the scenery such as forests, mountains, lakes, or on the people. Visualize the people in the place one by one and meditate on them.

You can meditate, in similar fashion, about a place you would someday like to visit. You can mentally transport yourself to the place and experience it, perhaps, in an even deeper way than going there. Later, going to the place is much more rewarding than it otherwise would have been. If you have a photograph or a painting, it can be used as part of the above exercise.

An interesting exercise is to establish a pattern of slow, deep breathing. After you have established this pattern, think of the number one as you exhale. Then take a breath and think of the number two. Do this until you have reached ten or fifteen. A variation of this that you can try in a later exercise is to mentally place the numbers beside and on top of one another in your stomach as you exhale. Keep them there and note how you feel once the mind has shifted to the center of your body. This is a classic Zen technique.

You may find meditating to a certain sound interesting. One way to do this is to listen to some music you like. Experience it, feel it, go with it wherever it takes you. You may want to let your body move with the music. This is often an exhilarating experience.

Many people like to chant during their meditation. A mantra is a sacred sound that, in some forms of Buddhism, is passed from the master to a disciple. In India the greatest mantra is om. It is said to represent God in all His fullness. To use this chant, think of om as divided into three separate syllables of equal length. Take a deep breath, and as you exhale, make the sound *owww* as in "cow," then slide into *ooou* as in "blue," and then into *mmmm*. Take another breath and do it again. Do this for a few minutes. Some people liken the effect to an internal massage. They also report calmness and expanded consciousness following. You may, of course, use other standard chants or develop your own.

Many people like to pray during their meditative exercises. Prayers should be focused on one simple idea or a short passage from a religious writing. Think about what this means and how it can apply to your life. In meditation one can develop a deeper inner communication with and sense of the presence of God.

Many other people find meditating on a poem or a line from a poem rewarding. A passage from a book can serve the same purpose. Many Oriental and Western writers who meditate have written of their reflections and experiences. These can be very useful as material for meditation and reflection.

You may want to meditate on a koan (ko-on). A koan is a seemingly nonsensical question that serves as a stimulus and focus for meditation. The word koan literally means a public document or a statement. It refers to a declaration that a master makes to a disciple for the disciple's instruction. There are many right answers to a koan, and yet there is no answer. The koan makes us aware of the limits of words and the depths of mind and existence. For example, one that has had considerable popularity in this country is, "You have heard the sound of two hands when they clap together. What is the sound of one hand? What is this sound for one thousand?"

Other such koans are: "Show me your face before your father and mother were born," or, "Where do we meet after you are dead, cremated, and the ashes are scattered around?" Another is, "All things are said to return to One. Where, then, is the ultimate home of this One?" Sometimes the koan takes the form of a command that is paradoxical as in, "Use your spade, which is in your empty hands," or, "Walk while riding a donkey." Many times they take the form of seemingly nonsensical answers to questions: "Who is Buddha?" Answer: "Three pounds of flax"; or, "What is the essence of Buddhism?" Answer: "My, what a large melon this is." One famous koan was for the master to hold up his walking stick in front of his disciples and say, "This is not a stick. What do you call it?"

Most of the exercises discussed above can be done in a half hour to an hour on a daily basis. It is not necessary to do them every day, but disciplined, regular use of them brings the best results. Beginners should not make the sessions too long.

For those interested in meditation, more information may be found in the public library or bookstores. The interested person may want to look into Zen, Yoga, transcendental meditation, T'ai Chi, and similar areas. One of the better basic books for beginners is *The Three Pillars of Zen* by Philip Kapleau, but there are many other excellent books available.

A word of caution is in order. Many people find meditation exercises beneficial, if practiced properly. But they can also be upsetting to some people. If you feel that they would be upsetting, don't do them. For those who do these exercises, it is best to start gradually and go only as far as you can with comfort. It is also best to work with and be supervised by someone with training and experience in this area.

One final relaxation exercise to be discussed is sometimes referred to as differential relaxation. It is very easy to understand and, with a little practice, can be readily employed. The basic point is that if we are sitting, standing, walking, running, or whatever, there are muscle groups that could be relaxed while the others work. We tend to tense and work many muscles throughout the day that could be in a state of relaxation. We do this because we typically involve our whole selves in what we are doing. Sometimes, though, we may be overdoing it. It is obvious that while sitting, many muscles could be relaxed. But even while running or walking, the arms, shoulders, back, and facial muscles, for example, could be relaxed. Analyze your daily activities and see how much relaxation can be worked in. Then discipline yourself to keep muscles relaxed rather than tensed when possible. Disciplining yourself is the difficult part. You will keep forgetting. One way to remind yourself is to paint a small red dot on the crystal of your watch. Then every time you look at your watch, you will be reminded to check and see if any muscles can be relaxed while you are doing what you are doing. If you learn to practice differential relaxation, you will see a general reduction of your tension and anxiety level, leaving you with a lot more energy and vitality at the end of the day. A physician, Edmund Jacobson, wrote extensively on the use of this and other relaxation procedures for the reduction of anxiety. He found them very successful with patients who are tense. A couple of his more helpful books are *Anxiety and Tension Control: A Physiologic Approach* and *You Must Relax: A Practical Method of Reducing the Strains of Modern Living*. Another physician, Herbert Benson, has written two very helpful books in this area, *The Relaxation Response* (with Miriam Z. Klipper) and *Beyond the Relaxation Response* (with William Proctor). Benson stresses the benefits of learning to relax for good physical health.

Remember, if you want to develop a physical strength, physical exercise is the way to do it. If you want to relax and reduce anxiety, the relaxation exercises outlined in this chapter can contribute a great deal toward that goal.

4

Straight Thinking

Many anxieties arise from thoughts we have or inter-pretations of events in our lives that we know, intellectually, should not be anything to worry about. We tell ourselves that a certain situation is not so crucial that there are many ways to look at it, and that it shouldn't bother us. And yet it does bother us. It can haunt and nag us daily, causing anxiety, irritability, and misery. Friends reassure us, and we tell them we know that what they are saying is true, but we still can't get our worries out of our heads. Sometimes, in cases like this, the main problem is faulty thinking. If we can think clearly and straighten things out in our mind, the problem dissolves.

A psychologist, Dr. Albert Ellis, has studied this aspect of anxiety for many years. He has developed a system of counseling and psychotherapy based on the idea of straight thinking. He calls his treatment rational-emotive therapy.

Often to make the technique of his therapy clear, he refers to the ABCs of emotional problems in the following manner. Generally when an Activating Event (A) occurs, it seems to cause an emotional reaction or Consequences (C) in a person. But on closer examination, we may find that A did not, in fact, cause C. What caused C was the Belief System (B) of the person. Thus, we have the ABCs of anxiety. We will get to D when we talk about the remedy for this situation.

First let's look at a couple of examples of how these ABCs can happen in everyday life. Suppose a person makes a mistake at work. That is A. That is the fact of what happened. Often this activates a Belief System that runs something like this, "I did a bad job today. Isn't that horrible? I *always* do that. I'm really incompetent at everything I do. I'll never succeed. I'm terrible. Most people know that about me. Probably nobody really respects me. I'll never be accepted or have any friends to speak of." The emotional Consequence of this, of course, is anxiety, depression, and loss of self-esteem. But, as Dr. Ellis would point out to such a person, this is *catastrophizing*. We are overreacting to the facts of the situation, and because of our faulty Belief System, we actually produce a catastrophic Consequence. This is irrational. If we could be rational about it, we wouldn't feel that badly at all.

Let's look at another example: Suppose a normal, average, likable teenage boy asks a girl for a date and she turns him down. This might activate a Belief System that says the following, "She doesn't like me well enough to go out with me even once. I must not be much of a man. All girls probably feel that way about me. This is awful. I'm a lousy excuse for a person. I'll never find the right girl to marry." Of course, the result, again, is anxiety, depression, and rumination about, "Who am I?" This is a common reaction among young adults and sometimes older ones, too.

If that were all that happened, it would be bad enough. But it usually gets worse. The person left anxious and depressed by this small event in life often finds that the reaction to the event is an Activating Event for other false Belief Systems, which cause additional emotional Consequences. The person continues in this way to dig a deeper and deeper hole, which he will never get out of if something doesn't happen to stop the process. Eventually this kind of process results in the person being preoccupied and distracted from meeting major responsibilities in life. He or she becomes tired and inefficient.

There is a solution, however. A person doesn't have to be victimized by these irrational Belief Systems. The answer is in learning to Dispute (D) them successfully. This calls for clear, rational thinking. Let's go back to the man who made a mistake at work that day. He could say something like this to himself: "I made a mistake today. Well, you win some and you lose some. Everybody has some good days and some bad days. The important thing in life is to *learn* from failure. Everybody fails and does a bad job sometimes. Nobody is exempt from that. The really successful people are the ones who learn from their mistakes and go back to do a better job the next time. Let me see. What can I learn from today? How can I do better tomorrow?" After some thought, he might say, "I feel better now. I think I''m going to get better at my job all the time."

Our boy who was turned down for the date might say to himself, "She doesn't want to date me now. Maybe she will some other time. There could be a lot of reasons for her saying no. Even if she doesn't like me at all, there are many other girls I can date. All guys—even movie stars are turned down—by someone in their lives. It's really a minor thing. Someday I'll meet the right girl, and we'll get along fine."

Of course, the points made in this chapter involve mental processes. They are intended to combat *irrational* Belief Systems that cause us anxiety, and a great deal of our anxiety is caused by just such beliefs. But behavior is part of it, too. Along with clear thinking, we need to be *doing* the right things and improving our actual performance all the time.

Many people find information to Dispute irrational Belief Systems by reading autobiographies of well-known people. It often helps eliminate irrational beliefs if we learn that others, even very famous people, have had the same thoughts or feelings that we have had from time to time. It also helps to discover that the same kinds of problems and events occur in such people's lives. For example, Louis Pasteur failed the admission exams for the University of Paris and did not get admitted on his first try. Even after he got in, he was regarded as a rather mediocre student and something of a plodder by his professors. Albert Einstein once failed an elementary math course. Thomas Edison was expelled from school as uneducable. Dwight Eisenhower was a constant discipline problem at West Point and was almost expelled on more than one occasion. Johnny Unitas was cut from the Baltimore Colts the first time he tried out. One could go on, with an endless list of authors who got hundreds of rejection slips before ever getting anything in print, artists who weren't recognized until after they had died, and so forth. The important thing to remember is that all people have setbacks. These events don't have to have catastrophic consequences if we think rationally about what has indeed occurred and what it means. These events can be a stimulus for growth and improvement if we see them as such, rather than provoking anxiety that leads to deterioration.

In analyzing Western culture, Ellis once identified twelve ideas that are very prevalent but that are stupid, irrational, and lead to problems in our thinking.

1. We must be loved by everyone, and everyone must approve of everything we do. This leads to much irrational concern on our part, especially when there are signs that somebody, anybody, doesn't like us or disapproves of something we are doing. This is a stupid position to take because it is not possible for everyone to like us. Nobody can please everybody. The very things that make one liked and approved of by one person make him or her despised by another. To try to be loved by everyone only makes a person less self-directing, more insecure, and less interesting. It is desirable to be loved, and it is necessary to be sensitive to feedback from others in order to relate to them better; but you should not try to be loved by everyone. Rather, you should actively seek out other people with similar interests and values so that you will get along well with them. It is better to spend our energy selecting and cultivating real friends than trying to please everybody and anybody.

In counseling young people, I frequently find that while they are in the public school system, they often feel that they want to be popular with everyone at school. This creates a very great problem. The range of interests, socioeconomic levels, family backgrounds, and so on, are so great that this is impossible. Yet they are thrown in with this large group every day, and they want to be approved of by them. The problem frequently diminishes after they get out of school because they can selectively associate with people of tastes and values similar to their own.

In general, it is best to maintain our own personal integrity, being true to our own values, while striving to be loving, creative, productive, and contributing individuals. If we do that, we can let people like us or not as they choose and not be overly anxious about it. We will have more real friends and be less plagued by irrational anxiety if we do so.

2. We must be thoroughly competent, adequate, intelligent, and achieving in all possible respects. It is obviously not possible to be perfect at everything. It is even impossible to be really *perfect* at anything. A person who adopts such standards is constantly full of anxiety about past failures to achieve perfection and the possibility she will fail to achieve perfection in the future. Even when one is acknowledged by others as being the best in an area (note that this is not the same as being *perfect*), such a person is continually anxious because tomorrow she may fall from this position. The person may decline, or a new and better challenger may appear. People with this irrational fear of failure often achieve a lot, especially in the short run, but they generally don't enjoy it. Often the methods they use to achieve their success alienate others. In the long run, many such people do not really achieve their full potential because of their faulty Belief System. It is best to realize that we are not, and will not be, deities. We can't be more than human. Nobody, including ourselves, should expect that of us. We should strive for achievement and accomplishment. But we should do this in the sense of making progress, learning, and growing as we live. We must Recognize all the time that as humans we will make mistakes; we will fail; we will have faults; and we will be subject to limitations and frailties. We won't be perfect, but we will do what we can and will improve as we go along. That is all anybody has a right to ask of us.

3. Certain acts are wrong or wicked or villainous, and people who perform them should be severely punished. There are no absolute rights or wrongs. There are things other people do that we wouldn't do; things they do that we consider inappropriate or antisocial; and things we wish they wouldn't do. Yet these people are not bad people.

Simply blaming them does no good. Punishing them does little, if any, good and often does harm. If we analyze why they did something, we can almost always see the sense of it from their point of view. Thus, their actions could be expected. If they were "wrong" (at least as we view things) in what they did, it is generally due to stupidity, ignorance, or emotional disturbance; so we should be very tolerant of their behavior and try to educate, redirect, and help them change to more desirable behavior. If we do so, we all come out ahead in the end.

Likewise, we should give ourselves the same break. If someone doesn't like what we do, we should not become anxious or upset about it. We should recognize that, within their framework, our behavior seems inappropriate. We should not be blamed for that. Nor should we become anxious and depressed about it. The rational thing to do is to compare ideas, discuss them, and see if we can learn from the experience. One or both of us may change, or we may agree to disagree, but we do better that way than by engaging in blaming and mutual hostility over a period of time that leaves us both losers.

4. It is a terrible catastrophe when things are not as we would like them to be. It is silly and childish when we think about it clearly, but many times we do proceed with the implicit assumption that the world and everything in it should be just the way *we* want it to be. We are deeply offended and outraged by all signs that it is not so. With all the different kinds of people in the world, however, it could not possibly be to everyone's liking. Also the harsh reality of the universe is that it was not created only for our pleasure and to revolve around us personally. Therefore we have to accept that the world, even our corner of it, will never be exactly the way we would like it. We should not expect it to be. When we see something we don't like, it does no good to perceive it as a personal insult or an attempt to defeat us. What we should do is say, "That is too bad," or, "I don't like that," and then try to do something constructive to change or improve it. As someone has said, if you are unavoidably dealt a lemon in life, you may as well make some lemonade. On the other hand, if it can't be improved at all, then we should resign ourselves to accepting it, realizing that this is sometimes the nature of things. We often tell our children that they have to realize that they can't have everything they want. Sometimes, though, as adults we make the same error in more subtle, sophisticated ways. When we do, it can only lead to unnecessary upset and anxiety.

5. Unhappiness is the result of external events and happenings that are forced on us and that we have no control over. Actually 99 percent of the unhappiness we experience is not caused by the unpleasant aspects of real-life events but is created internally by the things we say to ourselves about those events. We can control the external events to some extent, and we can learn to control our internal responses to these events almost completely. For example, if I lose my wallet with $1,000 in it, I may become very anxious, depressed, and unhappy about it. The actual event, however, is *not* that bad. It will take me maybe an hour to notify my credit card companies and the various governmental agencies. I will have to buy a new wallet, and I lost $1,000. Viewed in terms of a lifetime, the loss of the money and time are, in fact, very small. But by overreacting, I make it worse and exaggerate its significance. We actually defeat ourselves by our internal reactions. The external event, if viewed rationally, would be a matter of only minor concern. We can often see the truth of this when someone else is involved. We often say, "I wish I had his problems," or "I wish that were my main problem." We also need to see the truth of it in our own experience.

6. We should be greatly concerned about dangerous and fearful things and must center our thinking on them until the danger has passed. This is irrational because such thinking will not prevent the thing from happening. In some cases, it even makes it more likely to happen. In other cases, we become so exhausted from worrying that when it happens we are less able to cope than if we had not worried so much. Also the large majority of what we worry about never occurs, or if it does, it is not as bad as we had expected. The best thing to do is face such situations head-on. We should strive to make them nondangerous and to handle them successfully when they happen, but excessive worrying about them serves no purpose. Even if the worst occurs, we should regard it realistically as an unpleasant event, one that we didn't like, and go on from there. We need to stop telling ourselves that every problem is a terrible thing and that it is the precursor of the end of the world. It is not.

7. It is easier to avoid difficulties and responsibilities in life than to face them. When we try to avoid difficulties and responsibilities, we create only more and worse problems in the future. It is best to face problems squarely and to solve them to the best of our ability. Putting them off only increases anxiety, depression, and guilt. Facing them increases our feelings of self-confidence, self-esteem, and happiness. The enjoyable life is not one without problems; it is one where we solve problems successfully.

8. We need someone or something stronger than ourselves to rely on. Nobody is completely independent, and we should have no fear of being dependent on others to some extent, as they are on us. We should realize, however, that this dependency is a matter of all human beings needing others. It is not so specific that we must have one certain person to be dependent on. If one person fails us or is unavailable, there are other people who can help. Our whole life is never dependent on one other person. Sometimes we may think it is, but it isn't. Life goes on with or without any one individual. On the other side of the coin, we need to develop our own integrity, independence, individually, and self-expression so that the failure or loss of someone close to us is not devastating.

Being overly dependent on another robs both us and them of the best in life. We become insecure and fail to learn and to grow. They are, in turn, burdened with us and cannot reach their full potential.

A part of this dependency is often expressed as a feeling that people owe us things because we did something for them once or that we are obligated to them for something they did. Neither of these is true. If we want to do something for someone, we should do it, and there should be no strings attached. We should expect nothing in return, except the gratification that we did what we wanted to. Likewise we should not feel obligated to others under similar circumstances. It is stupid and irrational to suffer anguish because somebody returns nothing, or even ill, for our kindness. This does not preclude, or course, striking a clear bargain where the terms are stipulated and understood by each party at the time. We do "give to get" on occasion But we also should give a lot just because we want to give, expecting nothing in return. If we do, we'll get our share, in the long run.

9. Because something greatly influenced us in the past, it must determine our present behavior; the influence of the past cannot be overcome. This is not true at all. While it is often difficult to change previous learnings, it is not impossible. The essence of life is growth and development. We never stop changing. We are not the same person we were ten years ago. The world and our circumstances are not the same either. We need to learn from past experiences but not be overly attached to them. What may have been necessary and appropriate in the past may not fit or work at all in the present. The rational person develops and improves throughout life.

10. What other people do is vitally important to us, and we should make every effort to change them to be the way we think they should be. Actually, other people's lives, problems, and behavior are their own business and generally no concern of ours. We really cannot control or change them very much. Efforts to do so backfire more often than not and only serve to worsen the situation. In general, we should strive for the utmost tolerance: to live and let live. Often we are generally more upset by the implications or interpretations we think are involved in their behavior than by the behavior itself. Usually the supposed implications and interpretations are not in the other person's mind at all. If the other person asks us for help and we want to give assistance, we may. Yet we have no reason to force our ''help'' on those who don't want it. If their behavior directly affects us, we may want to discuss it with them and seek a solution. But many times we may just have to learn to live with the situation. A professor of psychology in my freshman year at college used to repeat in his lectures, ''We may as well learn that people have faults and decide to live with them anyhow.''

11. There is one perfect solution to every problem, and if it is not found, the result will be terrible. This is irrational because there are many possible solutions to most problems, but seldom is there any perfect solution. Each alternative solution has some good and some bad features. All we can really do is select one of the better alternatives and give it a try. If it doesn't work, we must try another. We live by doing the best we can in any set of circumstances. When we do this consistently, things seem to go well and catastrophies do not really beset us on every side. To hold out for perfection only causes needless anguish and often leads to worse solutions in the long run. If we hold out for perfection, decisions are often made by default. Seldom are these the best ones.

12. You have virtually no control over emotions; you are their victim, and you cannot help how you feel. In reality, we can exert a great amount of control over our feelings in many ways. If we work at it, especially through rational thinking, we can learn to control our emotions rather than being controlled by them.

Ellis later added more irrational ideas to the above list and eventually concluded that there are three major categories of irrational thinking under which these specific ideas can be classified.

1. *I* must perform well and/or be approved of by significant others, or else *I* am an incompetent, unlovable person.

2. *You* must treat me kindly and fairly, or else *you* are a rotten, damnable individual.
3. *Conditions* must be favorable and fortunate (bringing me much gain and little pain), or else life is terrible, I can't stand it, and it is hardly worth living.

Thinking about the above types of irrational thinking and employing the alternative principles of rational thinking protects us from much needless anxiety. Some people have found it helpful to get together with a friend or a group of friends and go over the principles of irrational and rational thinking together. Each can share experiences and examples of the principles and encourage the others to think and live rationally. As the reader may have noted, many of the rational principles are drawn from Stoic philosophy. Those interested may want to read more of the Stoic philosophers. Some of Ellis's books are also very helpful, such as *A New Guide to Rational Living* (with Robert A. Harper) and *Growth through Reason*. Another book that is useful, though written mostly for depressed people, is *Feeling Good*, by David D. Burns.

Approaches similar to the above have been developed as a system of psychotherapy by psychologists and psychiatrists. For example, Aaron Beck has published a book (with Gary Emery and Ruth Greenberg) entitled, *Anxiety Disorders and Phobias: A Cognitive Perspective*, to help mental-health professionals use these ideas with patients.

5

Existential Anxiety and Creative Living

IT is almost trite to comment on the rapid tempo of change in society today and on the growth of knowledge, technology, and affluence, but the fact is that the pace has quickened in the last generation or two. As someone has quipped, "If it works, it's obsolete." The world is literally changing so rapidly that children today are born into a world that will no longer exist when they are adults. They will be educated in school for tasks that shortly after they graduate will no longer have to be done. In years gone by, things were more stable and predictable. The struggle for survival seemed to give intrinsic meaning to life, and goals seemed obvious. With the technology and affluence of today, however, mere survival is no longer much of a struggle for most people in our country at least. In such circumstances, people begin to take stock of the meaning and *quality* of their existence. When they do, they often find themselves completely perplexed by questions such as, "Who am I? Where am I going? Why? What does it all mean? Does it really matter?" Intense anxiety and much anguish often accompany these questions.

Some psychotherapists have developed what is called existential psychotherapy to help people deal with these questions and problems. One of the more interesting pioneers in this field is the Viennese psychiatrist Viktor Frankl. Dr.

Frankl sometimes asked a despairing patient, "Why is it that you do not commit suicide?" With that jolting thought, he was able to find a small corner to begin helping the patient find a meaning for life.   Frankl is well qualified to comment on the meaning of life. His ideas were tested when he was a prisoner in a German concentration camp during World War II. One of his early books was entitled *From Death Camp to Existentialism* (later revised and published as *Man's Search for Meaning*), and it led some people to think he originated his ideas in the camp. He once told me, however, that he had developed his ideas and had a manuscript for a book describing them before he was taken to the prison camp. His ideas were tested in the camp, and he emerged more convinced than ever.

Frankl believes that the main motivation of human beings is to discover the meaning of existence. He refers to this as the will-to-meaning and contrasts it with the two other prevalent notions about the nature and motivation of humans. One is that we are motivated by seeking pleasure and avoiding pain. This hedonistic view is termed by Frankl the will-to-pleasure. It is endorsed by many in different fields. In psychiatry, Sigmund Freud was one of the main exponents. The second is the idea that humans are driven by a desire to master and conquer. This view was proposed by Alfred Adler among others and is characterized by Frankl as the will-to-power. Frankl thinks that these latter views, while containing a grain of truth, are misconceptions if we are seeking the main motivating force in humans. The main force is the drive to understand the meaning of existence. This is what separates Homo sapiens from other animals. Animals seek pleasure and conquest, but meaning is unknown to them. The essence of humans is meaning.

When one's will-to-meaning is thwarted, Frankl refers to this as existential frustration. This existential frustration grows out of an existential vacuum in the person's life and manifests itself mainly in a state of boredom. There is a feeling of emptiness, a void within oneself, and the feeling that nothing is worthwhile. This state of boredom and void is not mental illness in and of itself. It is a "dis-ease" of the spirit and is common to all people until they resolve it by discovering meaning in their existence. If it persists, however, it is a fertile breeding ground for anxiety, neuroses, and other emotional problems.

Neuroses and emotional disturbances can, of course, arise from other causes, but today a large number of them develop out of existential vacuum and frustration. These are referred to by Frankl as *noogenic neuroses*. This word is made up of the word *noos*, which, in this context, means "spirit," "soul," or "mind," and *genic* which refers to "origin" or "beginning." They are neuroses that develop out of the problems of the spirit. Of course, even the other neuroses have an existential dimension in that they involve the spiritual dimension in one way or another. According to Frankl, a person cannot make life meaningful nor can anyone else give one meaning for life; one must discover it. Others can help with this discovery. Frankl calls the system of psychotherapy that he has developed to do this *logotherapy*. In this context, *logo* or *logos* refers to "meaning." The treatment helps the person discover meaning. Frankl is fond of quoting Nietzsche to the effect that one who has a *why* to live for can bear almost any *how*.

Many of the ideas and techniques that Frankl has developed can be used to help deal with the anxieties we often feel in life. Frankl points out that basic to being human is being conscious of and faithful to our responsibilities in life. Living our lives in such a way that we are responsible toward ourselves and toward others is the meaningful life. This is an ongoing process, not a status that we reach. Humans are not content when they reach homeostasis, or equilibrium, where all pressures are absent. They are most content or happy, and life is most meaningful, when one is responsibly meeting and solving problems.

Life also has meaning when one is growing and progressing toward the achievement of values. There are three main areas of these values: creative, experiential, and attitudinal.

Creative values are realized when one works for the benefit of society. When we think of creative contributions, we generally think of such things as art, music, and literature. These are included in what Frankl means. A person seeking to realize such values might want to take up one of these endeavors as a pastime or a profession. Most community colleges have courses that can get one started in them. The library, of course, has a wealth of information on such areas. There are also individuals and clubs in every community that can facilitate a person becoming creative in everything from painting to wine making or woodworking. Such achievement provides part of the meaning of life.

Creative values, however, are much broader than this. For example, doing a good job at our work and being proud of our product, whatever it may be, are creative values. If we approach our daily jobs as a vehicle for expressing the creative values in life rather than putting in time to get a paycheck, we will discover a real and exciting dimension of existence that is all too often missed in the zombie like work world. When we approach our work in such a manner, everyone profits. We have richer lives, and we enrich the existence of those around us.

Creative values can be expanded even further. We can give of ourselves to others—friends, family, and neighbors. Putting a Band-Aid on a child's skinned knee and offering comfort is a very creative act. Working in community projects also can be. In responsible achievement, we find one of life's real meanings.

The second area is that of experiential values. This has to do with simply experiencing and appreciating such things as love, joy, curiosity, knowledge, nature, music, art, and history. Seeing the good, true, beautiful, interesting, and exciting in life leads to the discovery of depth and meaning. We do this by going to places where things are happening and becoming a part of them. We can attend concerts, visit art galleries, go to plays. Athletic events, if properly viewed, are a thrilling art form. Travel, reading, and a host of other activities could be included. There is an old joke about the man who spent a month one weekend in Waco, Texas (where the author lived when these lines were originally written). For a person who experiences and appreciates life, however, such a weekend could be an exciting adventure. Experiential values can also be realized by knowing a person in all of his uniqueness. Talking with and getting to know other human beings can be a remarkable experience if real communication occurs.

Attitudinal values have to do with facing life with the right attitudes. For example, if we can avoid suffering, we should; but if we are faced with unavoidable suffering, this can be a positive force in our lives. Suffering is ennobling if it is for a purpose and we bear up under it with strength. If our suffering contributes to another person or to an important cause, we are privileged to bear it. In one of his writings, Frankl tells of an old man who was despondent because his wife, whom he loved very much, had died. Frankl told the man that he was very happy for him. The man replied, "How can you say that?" Frankl went on to point out to him that if he had died first, his wife would have known the grief. But because she had died first, he was privileged to bear the grief for her.

We also learn from suffering. Tribulation is a great instructor. The carefree life may be good, but the lessons of suffering lead to a personality of much greater depth and quality. Suffering can be a strong stimulus to growth and development. Thus, real meaning in life can often be found in suffering.

Another attitudinal value has to do with one's view of happiness. Frankl has characterized the United States as being afflicted by "fun morality." We feel that the basic value and goal in life is to be happy and to have fun. This robs us of the significance of suffering in life because when we suffer we feel doubly bad. We feel bad because of the suffering, and also we feel ashamed and bad because of our unhappiness. The right attitude toward happiness, however, is that it is not to be sought after, or even expected, all of the time. It is a by-product of living our lives in such a way that we fulfill their meaning and attain positive values. This is true happiness as opposed to fun.

Another attitudinal value concerns time. In his book *The Doctor and the Soul* (New York: Alfred A. Knopf, 1972, 2nd ed., pp. 33–34) Frankl includes the following comments on time:

> Time that has passed is certainly irrecoverable; but, what has happened within that time is unassailable and inviolable. Passing time is therefore not only a thief, but a trustee. Any philosophy which keeps in mind the transitoriness of existence need not be at all pessimistic. To express this point figuratively we might say: The pessimist resembles a man who observes with fear and sadness that his wall calendar, from which he daily tears a sheet, grows thinner with each passing day. On the other hand, the person who takes life in the sense suggested above is like a man who removes each suc-

cessive leaf from his calendar and files it neatly and carefully away with its predecessors—after first having jotted a few diary notes on the back. He can reflect with pride and joy on all the richness set down in these notes, on all the life he has already lived to the full. What will it matter to him if he notices that he is growing old? Has he any reason to envy the young people whom he sees, or wax nostalgic for his own youth? What reasons has he to envy a young person? For the *possibilities* that a young person has, the future that is in store for him? "No, thank you," he will think. "Instead of possibilities, I have realities in my past—not only the reality of work done, but of love loved and of suffering suffered. These are the things of which I am most proud—though these are things which cannot inspire envy."

Your attitude toward your role in life is similarly important. Everyone has a unique destiny and contribution to make in life that nobody else can make. It is your responsibility to find that role and your duty to carry it out. Doing so gives meaning to life. Death also gives meaning rather than destroying it. If life were not finite, everything could be put off until later. There would be no need for us to be active, to do, to accomplish. The fact that life must end makes the present significant. Thus, death is a part of life. It is sometimes interesting to approach a new day as though you were living it for the second time and had done it wrong the first time, as you might this time, had you not thought about it in this new way.

Living a life that expresses itself in the ways outlined above results in a life that has meaning. The person does not experience needless anxiety because of existential frustration.

There are also some specific techniques that Frankl has developed that he uses with his patients. These techniques enable the person to put things in perspective and discover the meaning in their lives. One is called *paradoxical intention*.

Paradoxical intention is based on the theory that, in many cases, maladaptive behavior develops because a person is literally afraid of fear. That is, you think a certain situation will make you anxious, and then you become extremely frightened even about getting into that situation. This is called anticipatory anxiety, and it can increase to disabling proportions. The fear of being frightened by a situation and the fear of a situation develop into a vicious circle that makes one avoid the situation as vigorously as possible. Such a person becomes overwhelmed with anxiety and is almost unable to function if actually forced into the situation.

In using paradoxical intention in such a situation, you make the thing happen that you fear most in the situation. This, of course, is paradoxical. The pathogenic fear is replaced by a paradoxical wish. This technique takes the wind out of the sails of anticipatory anxiety, enabling the person to relax and handle the situation much more calmly. A humorous example of this is offered by Frankl. He tells the story of a very severe stutterer he treated as an adult. The man told him he had stuttered ever since he could remember. There was only one occasion when he didn't; it was when he was twelve years old. He hooked a ride on a streetcar and was caught by the conductor. He thought to himself that he would stutter and show the conductor that he was just a poor stuttering child. But when he tried to stutter, he was unable to do so.

Another example from one of Frankl's colleagues concerns a man who had had a heart attack. He became very afraid of any sign of change in the rate of his heartbeat and was afraid to leave the hospital for fear that he might need medical attention at any moment of the day. When one of his anxiety attacks started, he was told to make his heart beat faster, increase the pain, and get as anxious as possible. The nurse then left him alone for a while. When she returned, he said he couldn't do it. In fact, the opposite happened. He now felt calm. This encouraged him enough to get up and take a walk outside the hospital, something he had not done for six months. In one of the shops he started to feel his heart beat faster. He started saying to himself, "Try to feel even more anxiety." Again, he couldn't do it and actually became calmer. Soon after, he went home and returned to his job.

If you wanted to use this technique for fear of public speaking, you might think just before getting up to speak, "I'm going to get as anxious as possible. I want anxiety and stage fright to flow through and envelop my whole body. I want to tremble and quake; to perspire and turn red; to stammer and stutter. I will be so anxious the whole building will tremble with me, and I'll probably drown the audience in perspiration. One thing is for sure, if the water doesn't get them, the smell will. I'll be the world's champion. Number one in stage fright. Do they have an Olympic category for that? I will have the gold medal." Doing this will, paradoxically, make you calmer. It is important to ridicule the fear and use a sense of humor in deciding what you will say to yourself about the fear. This defuses the situation, making it possible for you to function quite effectively.

According to Frankl, paradoxical intention relieves existential anxiety because it calls attention to the way we often focus our attention on the trivial things in life and exaggerate them. This leads to irrational, unnecessary anxiety. If we call a halt to such nonsense and begin to concentrate on more meaningful things, we get rid of anxieties and live a more fulfilling, more purposeful, and happier life. Paradoxical intention is a way of calling the bluff on these trivial fears. Of course, such fears thrive in an existential vacuum. So living a meaningful life is good protection from them.

Another technique developed by Frankl is called *de-reflection*. De-reflection is somewhat similar to paradoxical intention. It is intended to counteract the obsessive-compulsive tendency we often develop toward self-observation. We begin by paying too much attention to something. The more we think about it, the worse the situation becomes. A good example is breathing. Try to watch your breathing and breathe normally. The more you try, the more your breathing becomes arrhythmic; the harder you try, the worse it gets. The same is true for insomnia. If you try to force yourself to go to sleep, you only ensure that you will stay awake. In the morning, when you give up because you have to get up, you fall asleep. It is possible to try too hard at some things, making success less likely than if we took it easier. In de-reflection the person is told simply to ignore the problem. Of course, many times this is easier said than done. It helps if we redirect our attention from the thing that is troubling us to some more meaningful value or something of importance. Once we do this, we often find that this resolves the problem. It no longer causes us undue anxiety.

Frankl contrasts the right and wrong approach concerning situations where these techniques are appropriate by talking about right and wrong passivity as well as right and wrong activity.

Wrong passivity refers to withdrawal from situations as a result of anticipatory anxiety. It is a flight from fear. Right passivity is the use of paradoxical intention. Through this technique, the person stops fighting the situation but is able to become involved in it without fear or anxiety.

Wrong activity is obsessively and compulsively dwelling on a problem or a concern until we are trying too hard and the goal becomes unattainable because of our overeffort. De-reflection is the right kind of activity in this situation. The person ignores the problem and redirects attention to more important things.

Some years ago Salvatore Maddi and Suzanne Kobasa became intrigued by the fact that some people break down under stress while others seem to thrive on it. They then had the opportunity to study a number of executives of the Bell Telephone Company. Through their research, which they reported in a book called *The Hardy Executive: Health Under Stress,* they learned a great deal about people who handle stress well. Many of these people have inherited a favorable physiological constitution to withstand stress. They also have good health practices and a strong social network of friends and relatives that provide support. Yet, of the greatest interest for our discussion here is the fact that these people also had a personality that transformed stress into motivation for effectively coping with situations rather than letting stress defeat and debilitate them. The personality factors that were associated with his hardiness in the face of stress were tendencies toward (1) commitment and involvement rather than withdrawal and alienation, (2) control rather than powerlessness, and (3) seeing things as a challenge rather than a threat. Frankl would, no doubt, agree.

6

Life Structuring and Engineering

★

OFTEN a lack of planning of our lives and the tasks we must accomplish results in our being subjected to many tensions, anxieties, and hassles. Fortunately many hassles are unnecessary and can be avoided very easily through planning. Planning may be thought of as structuring or engineering. In structuring, we give organization to situations and set things up so that they will go smoothly. In engineering a situation, we develop a plan or strategy of activity that will lead to a desired result.

Let's consider structuring first. Many times we are confronted with a task that puzzles us in terms of exactly how we should proceed. We don't know where or how to start. This leads to much anxiety and frustration. Often it results in our putting off doing anything about the task and eventually leads to failure. Frequently, if we can clearly structure the situation, we will get over the hump of inactivity. Then we have a good chance of successfully completing the task. For example, suppose our boss wants us to give a talk to a group of new employees at a dinner meeting. This is a rather vague request, and in many companies it might be communicated to a person over the phone or in a memo following a meeting by the committee planning the program. Such a vague request often leads to considerable anxiety about what is expected and what to say. We want to do a good job, especially in front of so many people, but we really don't know where to start. If we structure the situation carefully, however, the task becomes much easier. To accomplish this, we might tell the person making the request that we need a little more information to make plans. We would then ask a number of questions such as, "What will have been covered in earlier meetings with the employees? What function is the talk to fulfill? How long should it be? Should it be light and entertaining or a more hard-hitting pep talk? Are there any points that should definitely be covered, or is the content entirely open? Are there any copies of talks given in previous meetings?" Once answers to questions of this type are obtained, the task becomes more manageable. The simple technique of structuring the situation keeps us from foundering and gets us started in the right direction.

It is also important to consider similar structuring questions about tasks we assign ourselves. If we think about what it is we are trying to accomplish, it will often help us to carry out the task efficiently, without undue anxiety and frustration. The basic principle of structuring applies to all sorts of tasks. Take, for example, a minor repair job around the house. If we think about what has to be done, plan a little, and see that we have the correct tools and materials at hand, the job can be fun. It is often enjoyable to putter around at little tasks. Poor structuring, however, results in frustration, anger, and failure.

Another very simple example might be routine tasks that we must do every day. For example, many people lay out their clothes for the day before they go to bed. They can sleep peacefully, and when they wake up in the morning they can get dressed and ready without having to make a lot of decisions or having to look for articles of clothing. I myself find it helpful to put things under my car keys if I don't want to forget them. That way I can't leave without seeing them. These are very simple things, but they can greatly reduce the number of daily hassles we get involved in.

Another common structuring technique that some people use is to keep track of appointments and duties by writing them on a calendar marked with the hours of the day every day of the year. Calendars of this type are made small enough to carry in a vest pocket or to keep on a desk. Keeping such a book around the house or the office helps people structure their days and enables them to keep track of things. Other people find such a system too constraining. Using this method I often failed to write everything down and kept forgetting to look at the calendar until it was too late, and I used to miss some appointments. People like me find it works better to jot things down on small pieces of paper. I constantly make lists of things to do and write notes to myself about things I want to remember. I try to keep small pieces of paper handy at all times. They are on my desk, by my chair at home, in my wallet, by the bed, in my brief case, etc. When I need to make a note or a list, I grab one of these and write on it. I then clip them together and leave them where I will see them. I may put them in my pockets, in my shoes (so I'll see them in the morning), in my wallet (so I'll be reminded when I buy something), on my desk, and in similar places. Periodically, I sort through my papers, throw the old ones away, put the important ones on top, revise some, etc. People are often amused by my ''system.'' It is messy, but it works for me, and that is what counts. I virtually never miss a meeting or an appointment.

I remember reading about a professor who also used this system. Eventually his students caught on, and as a joke they began to write nonsense notes, which they put in his pockets and on his desk when he wasn't looking. He spent considerable time puzzling over what he had meant when he wrote those notes.

There are many other small structuring techniques that can make life more comfortable. Scheduling your departure for meetings and appointments with enough time so that you don't have to rush is an example. Of course, it is possible to get overly anxious about being on time. This is a mistake, too. It is best, however, to start out early enough to make it on time and establish a reputation for being punctual. Then, if on occasion you are late, you can take your time and not worry about it. Since you are usually on time, being a little late sometimes is easily forgiven.

While one can become overly compulsive about such techniques, life structuring can prevent many needless anxieties from ever arising. Thinking and planning in advance are the keys. If we do that well, the event will be no problem when it occurs. Often when I'm coaching a student about a public presentation she is going to make, I tell the student to be sure to have a closing sentence in mind for the talk. Otherwise, one may get to the end and discover there is no way to stop. The feeling of panic and growing embarrassment that develops as a public speaker in this situation continues to talk without making any further sense can easily be avoided by planning the closing in advance. The same principle applies to many other areas of life. Planning and structuring prevent anxiety. At the University of Oklahoma Medical School we train many students in the health professions every year. The demands on them are heavy as they fulfill all of the tasks assigned. Every year when the new students arrive our faculty write on the blackboard this message, "Remember, structure is your friend."

As I indicated at the outset, engineering of life situations is also very important in reducing anxiety. Engineering involves a more active process than structuring. There are many situations that are very frustrating and cause significant anxiety. With some forethought, however, it is often possible to engineer the problems out of the situation. A good example of this concerns the common problem of Sunday neurosis. Many people find their week very hectic and look forward to the relaxation of the weekend. Often the weekend starts out all right, and they do feel relief. By Sunday afternoon, however, they begin to feel depressed, anxious, and at loose ends. They just don't know what to do with themselves and feel miserable. They find themselves desperately wishing it was Monday morning so they could go back to work and get over their distress. This is, of course, very unfortunate because Sunday afternoon and evening can be a very enjoyable time. Most people do not relax nearly enough, and this opportunity should not be wasted.

A very effective way to deal with Sunday neurosis is to engineer it out of existence. The way to do this is simple. Plan some activity that you ordinarily enjoy but don't get around to doing very often and do it during that time. Take the family for a ride. Go to the beach. Go on a picnic. Invite some friends over to watch a football game or for dinner. Work on a hobby. Go to a concert. See a movie. Visit relatives. There are a thousand things that can be done. Doing these will make the week more enjoyable because you can look forward to them. It will make the weekend more enjoyable by helping you to relax and have some pleasant recreation. Make sure the activity selected is one that is relaxing, that you sincerely enjoy, and that adds a pleasant dimension to your life. Usually if you do this for a few weeks, the problem of Sunday neurosis disappears. At that point, it is not necessary to plan some major activity every Sunday, but occasional activities will continue to be very enjoyable.

Of course, if we frequently feel the effects of rather intense Sunday neurosis, and if our attempts at engineering do not prove very successful, it may be that there are some unresolved problems in our lives that we crowd out by keeping busy during the week. When we finally slow down, these problems surface and the feelings are depressing. If this is the case, it is wise to think about and work out solutions to these problems either on our own or with help from a friend or a professional counselor. Many times Sunday neuroses are not that deep or complicated.

Another example of engineering can be found in the area of entertaining. Most people are fairly adept at this and do a good job at engineering this rather simple situation. Yet many others have problems with it and become very anxious when called on to entertain guests in their home. Even those who do not have much trouble in this area may have trouble if the guests are unusually important or threatening in some way. Proper engineering in this type of situation calls for deciding what type of entertaining you wish to do. Is it to be a large cocktail party or a small, intimate dinner party? Will it be for old friends or for people who have not previously met? Once some basic decisions are made, you can begin to engineer the situation so that anxiety will be unlikely to occur. You need to consider the evening from start to finish and arrange things so they will go smoothly. For example, if it is to be a small dinner party, you may already know whether any of the guests have specific dietary requirements due to health problems or strong personal likes or dislikes. If you do not know, it is a good idea to check this with each guest. With this information, it will be possible to plan a menu. The menu might be one that involves food that is not highly risky in terms of the possibility of turning out badly and that can be prepared to a considerable extent ahead of time. The guests should be chosen so that they will enjoy one another's company and will be able to keep a lively conversation going. Structured activities such as listening to one of the guests sing or play a musical instrument can be planned to add to the evening.

While the above are only a few examples, planning of this type will have the effect of engineering anxiety out of such situations. It is better to engineer situations in this manner and keep anxiety from growing out of proportion than to avoid them or to endure them with great pain. After we have had some successful experiences, the planning and engineering will not need to be so elaborate. Much of it will become automatic, and we won't even have to think about it.

The same general point can be made about all of the suggestions made in this chapter. They may seem rather elaborate and overdrawn. But the point is that they should be used to reduce anxiety and hassles in situations that often upset us. If we don't need them in certain situations, then no purpose is served by using them.

We all have situations that just seem to be hard for us to handle. Structuring and engineering can often make them easier to manage. The exact situations that need that type of planning and the specific techniques used will vary from person to person depending on your life-style, what seems to work, and what you are comfortable with, but anxiety can be planned out of existence with proper structuring and engineering.

One of the most important areas in which these methods may be necessary is in time management. Most of us never seem to have enough time to do all the things we want. As a result, we go through life wishing we had more time for activities that we really enjoy, while spending a great deal of time on things that we don't enjoy. Recently there have been a number of articles and books written on the topic of how to manage time. When you think about it, time is certainly the most precious possession we have. Benjamin Franklin once said, "To love life is to love time, because time is the stuff of which life is made."

If we learn some of the techniques of time management, we will find that it is possible to get all of the work done that must be done and still have considerable time left for other activities. One of C. N. Parkinson's basic laws is that work will expand or contract to fill the time that one has to perform it (*Parkinson's Law and Other Studies in Administration,* C. N. Parkinson).

The first step in time management is to analyze everything that we do at work and at home each day of the week. We should consider for each activity whether or not we want to continue devoting time to that activity. A good question to ask about an activity is, "What will happen if I don't do this?" Most people can find many activities that they perform that don't really matter. If they don't really matter, don't do them. Do something that makes a difference. For the remaining activities, arrange them in a daily list in terms of priority. Each day work through the list as far as possible. Most of us will never get through the whole list in a given day. But, we will generally get through the top three or four. Those left over can be considered with respect to their inclusion on the list for the next day and their ranking on that list. By using this system, we make certain that we do the important things and do not waste time on unimportant activities. As we analyze our duties we may also discover that it is possible to delegate some of them. A good rule is to delegate any activity that you don't like to do and that is fair or reasonable to delegate. One of the most certain ways to waste time and be so exhausted that you cannot do the things you want to do is to try to do everything yourself.

Time management also involves becoming more efficient at everything we do. To become more efficient, we should think about each task that we have to accomplish and consider whether there is a better way to do it than we have gone about it in the past. Often we will immediately spot a better way. Other times we may need to ask those who seem to be more efficient than we are in that area. With a little thought, however, most of the things we do daily could be done more efficiently. For example, if we wish to shop for an item and compare prices, we can get in the car and go from store to store. Yet many items can be compared readily, at least initially, by calling each store on the phone to get a description of the product and the price. We may then only have to actually go and inspect two or three items before making our purchase, rather than visiting several stores that don't carry the product or have a product that is unsuitable. It is also possible to use the telephone in place of meetings or appointments. It is amazing that business that can be transacted in five to ten minutes over the phone will generally take thirty minutes to an hour if a face-to-face meeting is arranged.

Another example of efficiency that many people have learned is that if we get in the habit of cleaning up after ourselves each time we do something, it never takes several hours of cleaning to put our house or office in order. Likewise, it is possible to double recipes when cooking and freeze part for a later meal. This cuts down on cooking time.

Another part of efficiency is choosing the time to do a task and making whatever arrangements are necessary to avoid interruption until it is done. Someone once described her job as a series of interruptions, interrupted by other interruptions. Nobody can function efficiently under such circumstances. Schedule specific times for tasks, and resist unnecessary interruptions by whatever means possible.

One final time-management principle that has a great effect on stress is, "If a crisis happens more than once, it should be planned out of existence.'' Much time is wasted dealing with crises. Also, crises obviously increase our stress. Yet most crisis situations can be anticipated and their effect greatly reduced by planning. Emergency rooms in hospitals have all of the supplies and instruments necessary for specific emergencies prepared and packaged in advance. When a person is brought to the emergency room, the staff simply retrieves the appropriate packet and attends to the patient. If they began their search for the necessary items at the time the patient arrived, the result in many cases would be disastrous. A couple of useful books for those interested in more information on time management are *Hour Power*, by Lee Pierce with John W. Lee, and *The Management of Time*, edited by A. Dale Timpe.

7

Realistic Goal Setting

★

SOME people just drift along with the tide. They don't seem to have any goals. Their lives appear to lack direction. As a result, they don't achieve much. Often they are very capable and talented individuals. People who know them frequently lament the tragedy that they are not more goal directed and more productive.

At the other extreme are people who constantly set very high goals for themselves. In fact, they set such high goals that it is impossible to achieve them. These people are chronically tense and miserable because they are constantly failing. Every unachieved goal is a failure. Even goals that they achieve but which took longer to achieve than they had planned are regarded as failures. Such people drive themselves relentlessly. Often they accomplish a great deal, but they don't enjoy it. The fact that they didn't accomplish as much as they had wanted to as soon as they had hoped robs them of any pleasure in their achievement. After a time they find their energy sapped by this tension. They become disillusioned with their goals and frequently turn to cynicism and depression.

Both of the above types of individuals suffer from the same basic problem. They are unable to formulate realistic goals to guide their lives. Commonly the one who drifts with the tide either sets very low goals or does not set goals at all because of fear and anxiety. This person is afraid he will fail and knows that that will cause anxiety; therefore, he does not set goals. The second type of person sets goals that are too high. As we saw above, this also results in defeat.

In addition to goals being too high or too low, we can set faulty goals for ourselves. This, likewise, leads to disaster. When we do this, we find ourselves expending a great deal of energy and time to achieve something, only to find that it was not what we wanted at all. Sometimes it is not possible to detect faulty goals in advance, but often if we examine our values and think about the goal, we can determine whether we really want it. When couples come to me for marriage counseling, the subject of divorce frequently arises. Many times the partners are sure that they want a divorce. They think they could be happy if only they could get rid of their lousy partner. I ask them to think about it a bit and tell me how many things actually would be different and in what ways they would be different if they were no longer married to their partner. Sometimes when they do this they realize that they have been *blaming* their partner for everything unpleasant in their lives, but if they are honest, they realize that the real causes lie elsewhere. Divorce, in such cases, is a faulty goal; in other cases, of course, it may be a very legitimate goal.

The task is to set good, realistic goals for ourselves. If we do so, it gives direction to our lives, gives us a feeling of accomplishment when we achieve the goals, and helps us be successful, productive people.

To better understand the process of setting goals we need to understand that there are long-range and short-range goals. Long-range goals refer to major things we want to accomplish eventually in our lives. Short-range goals refer to the things we have to do more or less immediately; they are the tasks that we set for ourselves to accomplish each day. Long-range goals are generally achieved by accomplishing many short-range goals. For example, if we want to be a teacher in high school, this is a long-range goal. Short-range goals toward that end would include passing tests and completing assignments in the necessary courses in college, accumulating a sufficient number of credit hours, obtaining a college degree, and finding a job.

There are rules that when followed enable one to set good long- and short-range goals. The following rules apply to setting long-range goals. First, decide whether the goal is an appropriate one. Watch out for those that are too high, too low, or possibly faulty. Careful consideration of all relevant information will serve as a guide. It also helps to talk to others and learn from their experience. Get good advice from friends and/or professionals about whether this is a good, realistic goal for a person such as you. In the end, however, you will have to make the decision.

Second, make long-range goals that are general rather than specific. If they are too specific, we almost always set ourselves up for failure. If they are more general, we will find that they can be achieved in a number of ways, and we can be content with a number of accomplishments. It is better to set the goal of being an educated person and going as far as circumstances permit in college training than to make the goal obtaining a Ph.D. from Harvard with a straight-A average. It is better to set a goal of being a good contributor to community betterment than to decide that we must be voted the most outstanding citizen by some club and be elected the youngest mayor the city has ever had. Goals that are too specific almost always are frustrated and lead to a feeling of failure. Even when achieved, they are often found to be hollow and false.

Third, once a long-range goal is selected, carefully analyze it in terms of the exact short-range goals that must be accomplished to get there. Determine the path of short-range subgoals that is most likely to lead successfully to the long-range goal *for you*. There is always more than one way to achieve a given long-range goal. You don't have to do it the way somebody else did. You need to go about it the way that is most likely to lead to success for you, with your strengths, weaknesses, and personality.

Fourth, start working systematically on the short-range goals and *be patient*. Things that are worthwhile take time. Set up a time schedule that is realistic. Then allow yourself half again that amount of time before you begin to worry about not making progress. People with goals they want to achieve always underestimate the length of time it will take to accomplish them. This sentiment is expressed in the humorous retort to the old saying, "Rome wasn't built in a day, you know." The retort is, "Yes, but I wasn't foreman on that job." Things always seem to go slower than you had hoped. I remember one of my research assistants telling me one day that he had discovered a basic principle of research. I asked him what it was. He replied, "Things take longer than they do." The point is we must be patient with goals. Otherwise we set ourselves up for chronic frustration, tension, and anxiety.

The following rules are helpful in setting short-range goals. First, as with long-range goals, short-range goals should be realistic. They should be small and discrete steps toward the long-range goal. They should be things we can do more or less immediately and that will move us along toward the long-range goal.

Second, they should be more specific than the long-range goals. They should be sufficiently specific to enable us to know what we want to accomplish next and where we are going. Otherwise we will find ourselves standing around thinking that we want to get closer to our long-range goal but are making no progress in the right direction.

Third, our approach to accomplishing these short-range goals should be planned and organized in such a way that we have a high likelihood of getting them done. The ideas presented in chapter six can be put be to work here.

Fourth, if we fail at one of our short-range goals, we should not make more of it than it really is. We often catastrophize at times like this and behave as though one false step means we will never make it to our ultimate goal. This is rarely, if ever, the case. If we fail at a short-range goal, we should back up and try it again, or we should figure out an alternate route that will get us around the barrier. We should not let minor setbacks depress us. They are to be *expected* and *overcome*. They are all part of the process.

When you achieve a short-range goal, celebrate it. Celebrate liberally as you go along. Psychologists would refer to this as reinforcement or rewarding yourself for desired behavior. Whatever you call it, it is very effective. The celebration can be a small thing or something bigger. For example, if you are studying for an exam, you can put some nuts or candy or a soft drink on the table. The material to be studied can then be divided into very small units, such as pages, sections of chapters, or basic concepts. As each unit is completed, you can reward yourself with a piece of candy or a sip of the soft drink. It is important to keep the study units small and reward yourself with small amounts of the candy or drink frequently. Massive rewards after massive amounts of work are less successful. If you try this, you will find that studying goes a lot faster and is much more enjoyable. This basic idea can be applied to all sorts of tasks. It is a simple technique, but you will be amazed at how effectively it works.

Of course, the celebration can also be more major for

accomplishing a more important short-range goal or for the final accomplishment of a long-range goal. Thus, completion of a course or a semester might call for dinner at an expensive restaurant, a short vacation trip, or a gift for ourselves. Use of this approach makes getting there half the fun. People who arrange their lives this way enjoy themselves and what they are doing.

Once the long-range and short-range goals have been considered and established, it is best to shift our attention and emphasis to *process*. The goals have to be carried lightly. If we fix our attention on them too firmly, we will find ourselves so future oriented that we never enjoy the present—always going somewhere but never arriving. Looking forward too much to goals in the future makes us unhappy with the present moment and tempts us to make excessive sacrifices to get to our goals. When we get to those goals, however, we always establish new ones and begin the process over. In that way we never enjoy living in the present, because we are preparing to enjoy the future, and that future never comes. Goals are for direction and planning. After they have been established, we need to put them in the back of our mind and begin to concentrate on process. Concentrating on process means immersing ourselves in and thoroughly enjoying what we are doing now, not just as a means to an end but as an experience in and of itself. If we have our direction set by goals and throw ourselves wholeheartedly into the process of living and doing, we are most likely to enjoy our lives and achieve our goals. As in many areas of life, we can go too far in either extreme. It is the right balance that is most satisfying.

Of course, saying we are not going to think about our goals too much is easier than actually doing so. To keep the goals and process in perspective we need to be mentally vigilant and refuse to let ourselves become preoccupied with future goals. We can do this by working at being patient and by forcing ourselves not to think about them too much. If you have trouble doing this, there is a technique called thought stopping, which might help.

Thought stopping is an anxiety-reducing technique that is used to get rid of obsessive ideas or thoughts that sometimes run through your mind incessantly. Often these thoughts preoccupy you to such an extent that you can't seem to get them out of your mind. This can be very upsetting and anxiety producing. In using the thought-stopping technique, you are instructed to get the thought that has been a problem firmly in mind. You then signal the therapist, who shouts very loudly, "Stop! Stop! Stop!" This is repeated several times each session for two or three sessions. After a few times, you are instructed to say, "Stop," in your mind while the therapist says it out loud. Then you are told to say it in your mind when the thought occurs during the day. You are also instructed that after shouting "stop," in your mind, you should think of something or do something else that is absorbing and interesting. This rather simple technique is often very effective in ridding a person of obsessive thoughts. If you have this problem in any area, you might want to give it a try. You, of course, could use it to reduce preoccupation with goals. Simply have a friend play the part of the therapist and shout, "Stop," for you. Often, if the thought is only mildly obsessive, you can skip the part of having someone shout, "Stop." You can just say it emphatically to yourself in your mind and then say, "I'm not going to think about that now." Following this, think about or do something else.

Another technique that often works in helping us to keep from being obsessively preoccupied with goals is to write them down on a piece of paper or in a notebook. Just writing them down reassures us that they won't be forgotten and we need not be mentally vigilant about them anymore in terms of keeping them in our mind. Having them on paper relieves us of that. Many people get their notebook out from time to time, read over their list of goals, and fantasize or project themselves into the future. They let their minds wander and think about what it will be like when they reach certain goals and the things they will do along the way to achieve them. Such fantasies are useful because they keep us motivated and often serve as a type of planning session. Using such fantasy sessions frees us to think about other things in between.

One final word about goal setting. In setting goals, flexibility is a very important point to keep in mind. Goals, once set, should not be looked on as "musts." With time, circumstances change, and we change. What may have been a good goal when originally formulated may not be such a good idea at a later date. Therefore, it is necessary to be flexible and willing to change goals once in a while. This can be done as we go along, day by day. Or some people use the leisure of vacations to take a trip and reevaluate goals when they have more time to really think them through. Sometimes we reach an important point along the way toward our aim that can serve as an occasion to reassess the goal. We may choose to continue on, to change it slightly, or even to abandon it in favor of some other goal that now seems better. There is only so much time in life, and we can't do everything we might like. A friend of mine used to say, "We do what we do at the expense of something else we might have done." This fact makes goal setting and periodic goal revision crucial.

8

Assertion

ONE of the most effective ways to keep anxiety at a minimum in our lives is to deal with problems as they arise, without putting them off. If we put off dealing with problems, often something that would have been easy to handle grows in seriousness and gets out of hand. Nipping things in the bud is a secret of success that many highly successful people have learned to use.

Another problem with procrastination is that even if the situation does not really become worse, our anxiety about it often increases until what is actually a minor problem becomes a major *psychological* hurdle. In our mind it becomes a major problem.

If we handle tasks and problems as they come along, it stands to reason that we will have less anxiety in the long run because we will have fewer unsolved problems nagging us. Also we will be able to enjoy our other activities and leisure more because we have gotten the problem out of the way. For example, you may have a job to do that takes one hour to complete. It may be that the remainder of the day or evening is free for relaxation. If you do the job first and get it out of the way, you can relax completely with a clear conscience. You have the pleasure of knowing that the work is done. But, if you try to relax first, while planning to do the job later, you often will find that you are unable to relax.

The knowledge that the job is not done yet and that you will soon have to do it keeps you tense. I once had a patient who told me that life was a clam. At first I thought this was some sort of delusional statement; yet when I asked him to explain, he said, "You have to jump on it and pry it open to get the goodies out."

There is an old saying that the best defense is a good offense. While this is not always true, it works in many situations. Psychologists frequently refer to learning to take action in the right way and at the right time as *assertion training*. The idea behind this is that if we take appropriate positive action, we prevent anxiety from building up. Fear often results from a feeling that we are helpless. Doing something about a problem gives us the feeling of adequacy and success, which is an antidote for the helpless feelings that often accompany anxiety. Any kind of action usually helps somewhat. Appropriate action helps most. Many athletes and performers know that most of their anxiety occurs *before* the game or before they get on stage. Once they get into action, the anxiety leaves. Most of us have had this same experience in one way or another.

Often when we face problems head-on, we discover that they were not nearly as bad as we had imagined them to be in our anxious ruminations. Norman Vincent Peale tells a story about something that happened on his honeymoon. He and his new wife were alone in a secluded mountain retreat. Peale happened to hear over the radio that a dangerous killer was on the loose in the area. He immediately began to be afraid that his wife and he might be in danger. After a while, he heard a sound out in front of their cabin. There were footsteps on the front porch. They stopped in front of the door. Though very frightened, Peale decided he had to do something. With all the courage he could muster, he went to the door and threw it open. There on the porch was a small chipmunk! If we face them head-on, a lot of killers in our lives turn out to be chipmunks.

Some time ago, my neighbor was taking a trip and asked me to watch his boat while he was gone. Some vandals had been stealing motors from boats in the area. One night while he was gone, I looked out the window and saw two men trying to get the motor from my neighbor's boat. Without thinking, I went charging out of the house, pointed a finger at the two, and told them to stop right there. Fortunately they both got up and ran. After they were gone, it dawned on me that I was standing there alone in my pajamas pointing a finger at two men armed with wrenches and hammers. If they had not run, it would not have been much of a contest. The point is that pure, simple assertion will take you a long way. Appropriate assertion is better and will get you farther in the long run. We will talk more about appropriate assertion in the latter part of this chapter.

First, however, it is important to distinguish between assertion and aggression. Assertion is attacking a problem, standing up for your rights, or doing the right thing at the right time. We are simply doing what we believe to be the right thing in the situation, and we do it without malice. Aggression applies to a situation where our attack is mixed with hostility and malice. We often realize that we are going too far or are overreacting due to our anger, but we go ahead anyhow. Assertion is a mature, balanced, and fair approach. Aggression, generally, is an immature one that is often not fair.

Perhaps an example will serve to clarify the distinction in the terms we are using here. Suppose somebody does something we don't like. The aggressive response might be to confront that person in a heated argument and/or look for some way to get revenge. The assertive way would be to approach the person and honestly say that we didn't like what happened. We might then show a willingness to listen to her side of the story and to discuss ways to prevent the situation from occurring again. It is obvious that the latter approach will usually lead to a happier, less anxious life-style.

To develop appropriate assertive behavior as a way of handling problems, it is necessary to analyze the situation very carefully. We must first decide what the proper and appropriate way of handling the situation is. To do this, we must be very objective and carefully consider all the pos-sibilities. Often it helps to talk it over with a friend whose judgment we trust. That person can help us think clearly. It is, or course, crucial that we let the person know that we want help in determining what is the *appropriate* way to handle the situation. Otherwise that friend may try to show friendship by supporting us in whatever we seem to want to do or may suggest some highly idealistic way of looking at the situation that sounds good but won't work in practice. Once we have decided on the appropriately assertive course of action, we need to plan in detail how we can do it and then go ahead and carry out the plan. It is best to pick some easy situations in which to practice assertion and then tackle more and more difficult ones as we increase our confidence. It is also often best to start with mildly assertive behaviors in situations and increase the strength of the assertion over time. The important thing, however, is to determine the appropriate assertive response for a given situation, plan exactly how we will do it, and then go ahead and do it. After it is over, we can analyze how it went and, if nec-essary, revise our plan for the next time.

Let's look at an example of this. Suppose we have a job to do such as figuring our income tax for the year—a task fraught with anxiety and approached with excessive pro-crastination by many people. We might analyze the situation and decide that it has to be done; there is no way to get out of it. Putting it off until the last possible minute only increases the anxiety and makes it more horrendous in the end. We may then determine to take the bull by the horns, sit down, and start figuring out our income, deductions, and so on. Perhaps we will just work on it an hour the first night. We will then return to the task the next night and the next for similar periods of time until it is done. After we have gotten into the habit of handling tasks in a mildly assertive manner such as this, we may find that we can easily be more strongly assertive in the future. For example, we may find that we can sit down and do the job in one evening instead of spreading it out in small doses over several evenings. By practicing, we can train ourselves to handle situations in an assertive rather than a procrastinating manner.

Or take another example. Suppose you have a friend who borrows something of yours, say, a lawn mower, and fails to return it promptly. This causes you a lot of inconvenience because it is not available when you need it. A mild approach to assertion might be to tell the friend that it is fine to borrow the lawn mower and that you don't mind that, but you might go on to say that you would like it returned right after she has finished using it. Tell the friend that you may want to mow your own lawn, and you want it to be there in case you suddenly take a notion to cut the grass. You can, of course, say this pleasantly and with a bit of humor. If you do it right, your friend will not be offended, and you will get your lawn mower back. If the friend is offended by such a simple, appropriate request, this should be looked on as the friend's problem, not yours.

A slightly stronger form of assertion might come later (if the person failed to bring the mower back after your mild attempt at assertion) or if you simply decide that you no longer want to lend your mower. The stronger form of assertion might be to tell the friend that you have decided not to lend the mower out anymore. You can explain that frequently it is not there when you need it, that it is beginning to show signs of wear, and you don't want to have to put a lot of money into it for repair, etc. You should handle the situation with tact and humor, but stand your ground. It is possible that the person may resent it, but if handled correctly, it is unlikely.

One way to further reduce the possibility of the friend's being offended is to do something that shows you are not rejecting the friendship in turning down the request; you are only setting limits in an area where you think they are needed. The way to show a person she is accepted even though a request is rejected might be to invite the friend in for a cup of coffee while you talk or invite her to dinner sometime later or compliment the friend for something she has done. In this manner you tell the person that you still value the friendship, but you need to put some limits on the situation under discussion. A reasonable person will be able to accept and understand this.

From the examples above, it can be seen that assertion can be used in simple task-oriented situations and in interpersonal interaction situations. While the examples given are very simple ones, the technique works well in more complex and emotionally charged situations also.

Deciding what is the fair and appropriate thing to do in a situation is crucial in using assertion. After you have determined what action is appropriate, do it openly, honestly, and with tact and humor.

A good thing to do after you have asserted yourself is to analyze how it went, so that you can learn how to handle such situations better in the future. Following the analysis, you may want to reinforce or mildly punish yourself for what you did. If you feel you did the right thing, you should say to yourself, "I did what I thought was the right thing to do in that situation. That's good. I'm glad I did that. Maybe I'm wrong, but I did what I sincerely thought was right. That's all anyone has a right to expect." By doing this you reinforce yourself for doing what you did. You feel good and happy about it. If someone disagrees, you might say something like, "Well, I did what I thought was right. Tell me what you think and what you would have done." Then, without becoming anxious or upset, you will be able to discuss the other person's view and possibly get some feedback and information that will help you handle similar situations in the future. You can still rest secure in the knowledge that in the original instance you did what you thought was right, and that is all you can do—it is all anyone can do.

Sometimes mild punishment of ourselves may be in order. If we handled something badly, it does no good to pretend that we didn't. It is best to say something like, "Well, I blew that one. I should have handled it differently." We should philosophically accept the fact that failure is a part of life. The important thing is to learn from our mistakes and failures so that we can do better in the future. Everybody fails sometimes. The successful person is not one who never experiences failure, but one who learns something from each failure.

Often after we have decided to assert ourselves in a situation, we may have trouble figuring out the best way to do it. Or we may know the best way but doubt our ability to actually carry it out. If we are not sure how to handle it, we can use a technique that psychologists call modeling. It is a basic fact that we learn a lot in life from copying other people. This is what psychologists mean by modeling. We model our behavior by imitating what other people do, as many parents of young children have learned to their chagrin. The same principle applies in athletics. Coaches demonstrate techniques and encourage beginning athletes to watch the professionals use those techniques. Likewise we learn much from friends, teachers, and others just by seeing what they do and trying it ourselves. This can help us learn to be properly assertive. We can observe someone who asserts herself the way we would like to and see how she handles such situations. "You can see a lot just by observing," Yogi Berra once said. Later we can do the same thing in a similar situation that involves us. We may not be too good at it the first time, but with practice we can improve. If we don't have an opportunity to observe our model in all of the situations we are interested in, we can imagine how that person would handle it.

Earlier in this book, we talked about behavior rehearsal, which is practicing behavior before we try it in a given situation. That approach works very well with assertion. We can practice alone, possibly in front of a mirror. Or we can get someone to play the other part and help us. Practice makes us more skilled and better able to behave naturally when the situation calls for it.

Another aid to assertive behavior is reading some of the books on positive thinking. Such books as *The Power of Positive Thinking*, by Norman Vincent Peale; *How to Win Friends and Influence People*, by Dale Carnegie; and *Psycho-Cybernetics*, by Maxwell Maltz can be very helpful. There are a number of such books in the library and available as paperbacks in the bookstores. The books have one fault; that is, they lead us to believe that if we only have a positive attitude, everything will turn out all right. This is a little too simple. It often takes more than positive thinking. It may take the right circumstances, the right behavior, ability, help from others, and so on. All things being equal, however, it will go better if we think positively. Such thinking helps us make the best of most situations and facilitates success, even if it is not enough in itself to assure that success. Books on positive thinking often contain helpful hints on good ways to assert yourself and provide support and encouragement to go ahead and try. They are well worth reading if we keep them in perspective. There are also good books on developing assertion such as *Your Perfect Right*, by Robert Alberti and Michael Emmons; *Responsible Assertive Behavior*, by A. Lange and P. Jakubowski; *Don't Say Yes When You Want To Say No*, by Herbert Fensterheim and Jean Baer; or, *The New Assertive Woman*, by Lynn Z. Bloom, Karen Coburn, and Joan Pearlman.

9

Problem Solving, Decision Making, and Brainstorming

★

OFTEN acute anxiety develops when we are faced with solving a problem or making a decision. This can be true of any type of decision, but it is especially true if the decision is a very important one. We find ourselves struggling with the problem of deciding. One minute we feel one way, the next minute we feel the other way. We worry that maybe we will make the wrong decision. We wish there were some way to determine the right thing to do. The more we put off making the decision, the more anxious we get. We know that we must make a decision, but we don't know what to do. The tension becomes excruciating. We can't sleep. We lose our appetite and become preoccupied with the decision we have to make. Some people have this kind of difficulty with little decisions as well as big ones. Other people have problems making decisions in some areas but not in others. In this chapter we will present some of the ways to make good decisions.

One simple way is to sit down and try to make the process more concrete. Often we have a number of vague ideas, fears, concerns, and so on, in our heads, but because we have not really put them into words, they are very hard to handle. A good procedure is to sit down with a piece of paper. Draw a line down the middle and put the reasons for a certain course of action on one side and the reasons against the action on the other. Study the lists and try to weigh your feelings. Often putting the reasons into words clarifies our thinking. Seeing them on paper in front of us helps us weigh the alternatives and make a decision. Sometimes it helps to make the list and put it away for a while. Later when you come back, the decision may be very easy. Or you may add or subtract from the list and then make the decision. At any rate, this technique does help clarify your thinking and move you toward actually making the decision instead of thinking about it in a very vague, disorganized manner.

A technique for problem solving and decision making that was pioneered by Alex Osborn is called *brainstorming*. The process of brainstorming is very simple and very effective. It is basically a procedure for groups, but it can be used as an individual technique also. To use it in groups, get some people together who are interested and cooperative. Somewhere around five to ten seems to work best, but often two or three are adequate. Specify as clearly as possible exactly what problem the session is to focus on. Then start generating ideas according to the four basic rules for brainstorming:

1. **Critical judgment of ideas is ruled out.** Criticism and evaluation of ideas will come later. Criticism of your own ideas or of the ideas of other people is stifling and inhibiting of creativity. It is not permitted during the session.
2. **Free wheeling is encouraged.** Try to come up with wild, unusual ideas. Ideas that are new and different are wanted. After all, if more conventional or obvious ideas contained easy solutions, we would not be so stumped by the problem. It is often easy to take a wild idea and tame it, making

it a very creative and valuable solution to a problem.

3. **Quantity is what is wanted.** What is desired in
the session is quantity, not quality. The goal is to
come up with as many ideas as possible. Research
has shown that a larger number of *good* ideas
actually are developed when we express all ideas
that come to us rather than when we evaluate them
and express only the "good" ideas.

4. **Combination and improvement are sought.** As
ideas are expressed, each person should think of
ways to extend, revise, or combine them with other
ideas to produce still other ideas or combinations.
In generating and revising ideas, consider such
points as: What other uses could this object or idea
be put to in its present form (uses that have not
been thought of or tried before)? What uses would
be possible if this object or idea were adapted or
modified in some way? What would happen if we
maximized or minimized one aspect or effect?
What if we changed the order and did it in a different sequence?

There is good evidence that using brainstorming techniques produces excellent results. It seems that one person's
thoughts and ideas often stir another's associations, stimulating that person to come up with ideas and thoughts that
would not have occurred in isolation, and vice versa. Also
the social motivation and facilitation of being in a group of
people working on a problem enables us to work more
diligently and enthusiastically than we would on our own.
Finally, the stimulating effects of competition and friendly
rivalry contribute to greater productivity.

There is an old story about the community stew. One

person had carrots, another a potato, another a piece of meat, and so on. When they stayed home, they all ate a meager and unbalanced diet. But when they got together and put what they had in a pot in the center of town, there was enough for everyone to feast healthily.

If you want to use group brainstorming to work on a problem, get a group of people together who are as motivated and concerned about the problem as you are. They might be friends who have interests similar to yours. If the problem is job related, they might be people you work with or who are in a similar line of work. They might be family members if it is a family problem. Incidentally, don't hesitate to include children in such sessions. Often they come up with some really outstandingly fresh and creative approaches. It is interesting to brainstorm such things as income-tax deductions, ways to save money around the house, how to get a job at work done more quickly and easily.

While two heads are better than one, and groups do better at brainstorming than individuals, this does not mean that you cannot do it alone. You can. Just sit quietly and let ideas flow, following the same rules as above. You can do it at home, in your office, while traveling somewhere, or anytime. The main value of brainstorming is to generate ideas. One thing that hinders decision making is inhibition of ideas. This is often because the person has become too rigid. To be rigid in your thinking means that you can see only one or two ways of approaching a problem and are not able to look at it from different points of view. If one of the solutions you are able to see works, then everything is OK; if not, you are in trouble. Such rigid thinking often leads to anxiety over problems that can be solved easily if we can break out of the rigid mold in which we find ourselves.

As ideas are generated during brainstorming, it is best to simply write them down as they come. Later go over them and evaluate them. Then prepare a new list containing some of the better ones. After some study and thought, prepare a list with what you consider to be the best alternative at the top and the least desirable one at the bottom. That way, you can try the first one and see if it works. If it does, you have solved the problem. If not, go to the next alternative and continue in this manner until you find one that works.

Ordering the alternatives in terms of their desirability requires that you consider several features of each alternative. This is, of course, the hardest part of the task. You may remember the old story about the farmhand who worked very diligently for his boss. When he was in the fields, nobody could keep up with him; he could do twice as much as other men. In addition, he seemed to enjoy and thrive on hard work. One day when it was particularly hot, the boss decided to give the man a break. He went and got him from the fields and took him into the barn where it was cool and where he could sit down instead of working so hard. His job was to sort the potatoes according to size into three piles—small, medium, and large. At the end of the day, the boss came back and was shocked to see that his best worker was sitting dejectedly in the corner and had hardly sorted any potatoes at all! Puzzled, he asked him what the problem was. The man replied, "It's these damned decisions."

One of the first things to consider in ordering the possible alternatives is their irreversibility. There are some that you can try, and if they don't work, no particular harm will have been done. You can simply go on to another one. But some of the alternatives, once tried, make further solutions harder or impossible to accomplish. Such alternatives should generally be placed farther down on the list.

A second consideration is the amount of effort required for trying one of the solutions. If it is easy to do, it may be worth trying and should tend to be placed closer to the top of the list than one that is very difficult or that takes a lot of time and effort.

A third consideration is the risk involved. If an alternative is attempted, what are the risks? What are things that might go wrong, and what would be the consequences if they did? Obviously, risky ones will tend to be lower on the list.

Another consideration is the probability that the alternative will work. Some are long shots, and others are almost sure things. This needs to be taken into account.

Finally, keeping the above principles in mind, we must consider the ultimate payoff. If we try a given solution and it works, how will it benefit us?

Using these principles, we will find that they are combined in various mixtures in the possible alternatives. With some thought, we can order them according to our preference and start to try them. I often like to start with a long shot that doesn't take too much effort, will not be at all irreversible, and that would have a large payoff—if such an alternative exists. If you don't have a dream, it can't come true. But if you try for your dream, sometimes you will obtain it. If it doesn't work, however, I then proceed down the list. The solutions I put on the bottom are ones that require a lot of effort, are irreversible, are pretty sure of working, but tend to have minimal payoff. Different people may prefer different strategies, and we may have different strategies in different situations. The important thing is to have a strategy and to execute it.

Some people find it helpful to write out their list of alternatives and check them off as they are tried. Others just keep them in mind. Putting them down on paper often makes one feel better and facilitates clear thinking and action.

There are some additional principles of decision making that are well to keep in mind. One is that in the majority of the situations we face, *only we can really make the decision*. Relying on somebody else to tell us what to do will generally not lead to satisfactory results. As is often said, advice is easy to give but hard to take. If a group of people happen to be involved, we may want to make the decision by committee vote, but the majority of decisions that we face and that produce anxiety are matters only we can decide. We may as well face up to this and do so assertively.

Second, we need to realize that the process of decision making is one in which we will sometimes make what might be considered the wrong decision. Actually, if we follow the principles outlined in this chapter, it will not be wrong. We will have made the best decision possible under the circumstances. Sometimes, however, the outcome may not be what we wanted it to be. When that happens, we need to philosophically accept the fact that everybody wins some and loses some—ourselves included. The main point is to learn from each experience so that we can win more than we lose.

Third, it helps a great deal if we practice reinforcing ourselves after we have made a decision. To do this, we can say something to ourselves like, "Well, I made the best decision possible as the situation presented itself. That's all I could do. I did what I thought was right and that's what a person ought to do. I'm glad I did it. I fulfilled my responsibility." Later, if someone else has a different idea or if things don't turn out the way you wanted, you can be open to learning from the situation. You need not feel defensive or upset because you have already settled it within yourself that you honestly and sincerely did what you considered to be the right thing and you feel good about that part. If a revision is called for, you are free to go ahead with that as part two of the process. You will then also reinforce yourself for doing that. The point is that you are monitoring your own behavior and doing what you think is right. This makes you a person of integrity and self-confidence. You are receptive to feedback from others, but you make up your own mind. It is this balance that makes a mature, responsible person. If we are overly stubborn about our ideas, we are not fair to others. If we are overly dependent on what others *think* we ought to do in a situation, we are wishy-washy and lack personal integrity. This makes us anxious and miserable. Successful decision making takes a balance of responsiveness to feedback and internal judgment. The fulcrum is self-reinforcement.

10

Nutrition and Exercise

WHEN I was a boy going to school in Madison, Ohio, we used to have a grade-school teacher named Pop Ryan. He was about seventy years old but was in excellent health and full of vigor. He was a man of the old school and used to lecture us on the importance of maintaining good health and hygiene practices. It was the old "sound mind in a healthy body" theory. We used to snicker at him while eating excessive quantities of hamburgers and French fries, with a soft drink to wash them down. We knew our diet would have caused his hair to stand on end, but we regarded him as sort of a kook. It's funny, though, over the years, as I learned more and more about physical and mental health, I began to discover that Pop Ryan had something. I've found in terms of my own experience and in clinical work with my patients that physical and mental health often go together. When we are tense, anxious, and depressed, we feel physical pain and general malaise. Also when we are physically ill, for example, when we come down with a cold or the flu, we often feel emotionally upset, depressed, and anxious. Good physical health contributes to good mental health and vice versa.

Consider general nutrition. Food has special significance for many people. Since we are often comforted with food as children, we tend to associate food with love and security.

91

Thus, many people find that they eat when they are anxious or tense. Eating makes them feel better temporarily. It is interesting to note that certain kinds of food or food prepared in certain ways may have the same effect. For example, many people find that very spicy foods, such as Italian or Mexican dishes, tend to cause discomfort. This may be the effect of such foods on some people. I was reared on food prepared by a wonderful Italian mother. As a result, eating spicy foods actually has a calming and settling effect on my stomach. Some of my physiologically oriented friends tell me that isn't possible, but that's the way it works for me.

Various claims are made from time to time that certain foods such as organically grown foods or uncooked food, or some special diet such as a strictly vegetarian diet will result in better physical health and possibly improve mental health. Because many of these claims have not been thoroughly studied, there is no scientific evidence to support them at present. But research is going on in many areas related to nutrition and health, and this research is shedding new light on the nutrition's relationship to the brain's activities.

For example, one notion currently being explored is that many people suffer from "cerebral allergies"; just as one can develop a runny nose or a skin rash when in contact with a substance to which one is allergic, the brain can react to chemicals circulating in the bloodstream in a similar manner. We know that the brain is richly supplied with blood vessels and, thus, any substance in the bloodstream can potentially influence brain function. It is speculated that if one eats certain foods to which one has a cerebral allergy, this might result in agitation, anxiety, depression, or some other mental symptom. Unfortunately there is no scientific evidence to support this theory in the form stated.

What makes these theories plausible, though, is that there

are some very general relationships between ingesting certain foods and the function of the brain that have been known for some time. For example, excessive consumption of beverages with caffeine can produce nervousness, anxiety, and irritability. Likewise, some recent research indicates that consumption of foods containing carbohydrates can have a calming and sedating effect on an individual. While some very general relationships of this sort have been carefully documented, the vast majority have not survived rigorous scientific research. For example, there has been considerable research on the relationship between sugar and activity levels in children. The overwhelming evidence in this area is that, contrary to many claims made, sugar consumption does not produce hyperactivity in children. Nor do food colorings, products containing wheat, and most other claims of this nature. We may discover that there are subgroups of individuals who respond to certain foods in a manner different from other people. While this is possible, most researchers in the area of nutrition do not expect many dramatic findings of this sort. At present, trained nutritionists are cautious about making any claims for such eating habits until there is sound scientific support for them. What is important to remember is that nutritional deficiencies result in declining health and disease, which are often accompanied by mental and emotional symptoms of one sort or another. Therefore, a well-balanced diet certainly contributes to the general energy level, stamina, and sense of well-being in an individual.

Many rules for good nutrition that are generally endorsed by physicians and nutritionists are aimed at avoiding obesity. Since you were a child you've been taught to eat a balanced diet each day. A balanced diet is one that includes the four basic food groups of (1) milk, cheese, and other dairy products, (2) meat, (3) vegetables and fruit, and (4) bread and cereals. Almost any diet book on the market will caution you to avoid too many fried foods and excessive consumption of sweets, to eat more smaller meals rather than fewer large ones, and to eat slowly, chewing food carefully.

You should also make mealtime a time for relaxing. Rather than eating hurriedly, gulping your food, and conducting business during meals, try taking a walk, reading, resting, listening to music, or some such activity to unwind a little *before the meal*. Then sit down and enjoy a leisurely, relaxed meal. You'll enjoy the food much more, take the edge off daily anxiety, and reduce the likelihood of developing ulcers.

There is currently some debate about nutrition in the United States. Some say our food storage and preparation methods reduce the nutritional value of the food we consume. Others insist that we are the healthiest and best-fed people who have ever lived. Still others say that while perfectly adequate foods are available to Americans, their eating habits do not provide them with the proper selection to produce a balanced diet. Nutritionists say that following a balanced diet (that includes foods from each of the basic groups) will be quite sufficient for most people's good health. No further supplements such as "health foods" or vitamins should be needed. At most, one might wish to take one multiple vitamin/mineral tablet per day of the type designed for such use. There is a lot of faddism in this area. Physicians are quick to point out that fad diets, large doses of vitamins, and similar practices may be dangerous and harmful to some people. Therefore, if you feel you are one of the exceptions that requires some dietary supplement, consult a physician who is trained in nutrition. Many physicians are not familiar with this area, but your family physician can help you locate one who is. The doctor can examine you and prescribe the right supplement or medication for you, if you need it. Doing this will enable you to get exactly what you need in a safe, supervised manner. Experimenting on your own can be dangerous.

Exercise is also very effective in reducing anxiety. How this occurs is not entirely understood. Some say that it satisfies our innate need to engage our large muscles in physically aggressive activity. In primitive times we had natural outlets for this kind of activity, but in our highly civilized, sedentary, and confined life-style we do not. More recently, researchers have begun to discover changes in body chemistry following exercise that may explain our changes in mood.

Physiologically, exercise affects all the systems of the body. Circulation of blood and consumption of oxygen are increased. Body temperature rises. Metabolism is stepped up. Waste products are excreted more rapidly from the cells and are eventually eliminated from the body through perspiration, urination, and defecation.

Prolonged and intensive exercise tends to produce an increased level of lactic acid in the blood. Although an increase in lactic acid is usually associated with the occurrence of anxiety, when secreted during exercise, lactic acid seems to reduce anxiety and tension. This may be related to the fact that the body produces chemicals called endorphins under such circumstances. Endorphins act on the body much like morphine does, reducing pain and promoting a feeling of well-being. Endorphin production probably also accounts for what has been called runner's high. Individuals who run or exercise vigorously for prolonged periods of time often experience a state of euphoria that occurs long after the start of exercise, when one might expect the individual to be feeling extreme fatigue and pain. The natural endorphins produced by the body, no doubt, are producing a high that might be induced under other circumstances by ingestion of drugs. A very similar state is often achieved by individuals who engage in meditation and yoga. To date, there have not been scientific studies of endorphin levels in individuals who have reached states of euphoria by these means. It is clear, however, that endorphins play a major part in many of the experiences of well-being that are associated with exercise. Many people find that it is very worthwhile to meditate during strenuous exercise, such as running, or immediately following. Again, the release of endorphins may well facilitate the process of meditation. Books by Dr. Kenneth Cooper, such as *New Aerobics* or the *Aerobics Program for Total Well-Being,* both of which are available in paperback, can be very helpful in planning a program of the type discussed in this chapter.

Over a period of time, exercise increases vital capacity. Circulation and oxygen utilization are improved, and a larger exertion is required before lactic acid is produced. In this way, it is possible that exercise serves as a sort of anxiety-inhibiting mechanism.

Whatever its basis, exercise does have an anxiety- and tension-reducing effect. Studies have shown that people on regular exercise programs tend to be more healthy, have better vital capacity, handle problems better, sleep better, and cope with life in a generally more satisfactory manner. Over a period of time, people on such programs generally feel better, are more optimistic, and have a better self-image. Thus, exercise immediately reduces anxiety somewhat, and over the long run it tends to inoculate us against development of future anxieties.

Exercise, however, can be very dangerous if too strenuous or of the wrong type for a person's physical condition. In general, the older one is, the more cautious one needs to be, but youth is not guaranteed protection against injury.

Every year young people engaged in athletic activities suffer heart attacks, strokes, and other complications. Before beginning an exercise program, it is very important to consult your family physician for advice.

There are two basic types of exercise that can be employed to reduce anxiety. One is rhythmic motion. Walking, running, swimming, and bicycling provide rhythmic motion. Jogging has become a very popular exercise of this type. Cooper's aerobics programs are very good. As he points out, such exercise not only reduces anxiety, it also increases general health, aids in weight reduction, and helps prevent heart disease and various other disorders.

The other major type of exercise that can reduce anxiety is stretching. You may have noticed that people frequently stretch their arms above their heads in times of tension to help relieve discomfort. You can elaborate on this basic technique. For example, if you feel tension in the neck, take your head in your hands and gently stretch your neck. Then hold the head and chin and exert pressure downward, again stretching the neck muscles. If the back is tense, bend and stretch in ways that pull the muscles gently. If your chest is tight, make some stretching movements with the arms in various directions until the tension and tightness subside. Practicing exercises of this sort on a regular basis can be very beneficial. You can even ask your physician to refer you to a physical therapist for specific instructions regarding stretching exercises.

When I encourage patients to exercise for anxiety reduction, I generally point out to them that to do the most good the exercise should be a regular activity. Therefore, it should be worked into their daily routine. Many people exercise first thing in the morning. Then they take a shower and go to work. I had a friend who was a university professor. He used to jog from his home to the university. He had a locker in the gym where he showered and dressed for classes after he arrived. Some people exercise when they get home from work or just before bedtime. Most cities of any size have groups who get together during their lunch hour at the YMCA or at one of the commercial health centers. Some companies provide facilities for exercise. But whenever or wherever one does it, *regular* exercise is the key.

If you have other physical problems, exercise can be recommended by your physician or by a physical therapist, who can recommend specific exercises for you to work into your regular routine. For example, I have a shoulder that pops out of place easily and a back that was injured while I was in high school. Both tend to give me a lot of pain from time to time. I consulted a physical therapist and learned some exercises to incorporate into my usual program. When I do these exercises regularly, my shoulder stays in place and my back gives me no trouble. As fellow sufferers know, these are no small benefits.

Because many people can't get too excited about getting up an hour earlier to jog or about giving up their lunch hour to do so, I recommend that they choose a sport they like and play it regularly for exercise. Tennis, handball, golf, boating, and swimming are just a few sports that can help you to relax.

Be sure to consult a physician before you begin an exercise program. Then start out gradually and build up your endurance rather than trying to do too much too soon.

Many people find hot baths to be very relaxing. The heat from a hot bath increases circulation, accelerates the metabolic activity of cells, carries away waste products more rapidly, and relaxes muscle tissue. It is a purgative process. While the reason is not fully understood, pain is also reduced under these circumstances. Whirlpool baths are even more effective. Small whirlpool units can be purchased for home bathtubs, and most exercise centers have them. The whirlpool turbines circulate the water, adding gentle massage to the benefits of the heat from the water.

Some people find alternating hot and cold water to be very relaxing. First take a hot bath or shower and stay under the hot water for four or five minutes. Then turn the hot water off and turn cold water on for about two minutes. This can be harmful to some people, however, especially if they have any type of circulatory problem. Therefore, it is best to check with your physician before you try this.

Sauna and steam baths are other ways to enjoy the benefits of heat. If you plan to use sauna or steam baths, it is important to familiarize yourself with the equipment and use it properly. Talk to someone familiar with the equipment you are using and read the manufacturer's manual. In general, the rules for safe use of sauna and steam baths are as follows:

First, sauna and steam baths can be dangerous for some people—the elderly and people suffering from diabetes, heart disease, high blood pressure, as well as numerous other conditions. In addition, you could be in danger if you ingest alcohol, antihistamines, anticoagulants, narcotics, tranquilizers, sedatives, or other medications before a sauna or steam bath. Therefore, as with other activities suggested in this chapter, you should consult your physician before you begin. A phone call to your family physician will suffice. If you do not have a family physician, use this as a good opportunity to get a physical exam and discuss your plans with the physician who examines you.

Second, be sure to read and follow the directions of the manufacturer of the equipment or of the person supervising the equipment. Do not use the equipment alone. Someone should be around to help if necessary. There should be a window for them to check on you, and there should be a clock clearly visible so you will know how long you have been in. If you are a beginner, start out with just a couple of minutes, no more than five. Gradually increase to a level that feels good. Never stay in more than a maximum of twenty to thirty minutes.

Do not exercise strenuously before sauna or steam baths, and do not exercise at all while in them. Do not enter them for at least an hour after eating a full meal. Drink liquids before and after.

Proper use of sauna and steam baths will reduce weight (though it is only water loss and will return shortly), increase circulation, lead to muscular relaxation, and possibly improve and clear the skin. There is no evidence that they prevent or cure the common cold. They are not recommended for people whose sinuses are draining or as a cure for a hangover.

Massage can have a similarly relaxing and beneficial effect. Massage increases circulation and metabolism in the same way heat does, and it appears to offer additional advantages. The mechanics of massage force fluid out of the tissues, thus reducing swelling and pressure due to excessive fluid that sometimes gathers after trauma or exercise. Also, the mechanical stretching of the muscles and connective tissues tends to relax them and reduce pain. Massage must be done properly to be of much help. Most health centers, many YMCAs, and similar clubs have trained masseurs available. Physical therapists also, of course, provide massage. Generally, a referral from a physician is required before a physical therapist can see you, but this is not hard to obtain. In smaller towns, a nurse, physical-education teacher, or a trainer for school athletes can provide massage. Many find that a good massage reduces anxiety remarkably and makes a new person out of them.

My experience has been that it takes a lot of encouragement to get people to try the things mentioned in this chapter, but when they do, they invariably report that the techniques work and that they never felt better in their lives. These techniques appear to reduce anxiety as well as improve the general health and stamina of the person. A regular program can involve minutes or hours per day, but it appears to be time well spent.

11

Recreation and Escape

ANXIOUS people don't have much fun in life. When we are anxious, we suffer such mental anguish and physical pain that we cannot enjoy ourselves. It is also true that if we do not make many provisions for having fun, we become more susceptible to anxiety. These two mind-sets tend to reinforce each other, and eventually we get into a terrible rut. We are anxious so much of the time that we can't enjoy ourselves, and not enjoying ourselves tends to make us more anxious and depressed.

There are a number of factors that can trigger this cycle. Often it starts with very real tensions and problems that, if left unresolved, eventually get us down. Then we get into the anxiety rut. Paradoxically, sometimes we become so familiar with our anxiety rut that we are afraid to venture out of it. Other alternatives seem vague, unfamiliar, and possibly even more threatening. Sam Keen puts it almost poetically. In his book *To a Dancing God* (New York: Harper & Row, 1970, pp. 109–110), he records a dialogue he had with fear. Part of it goes like this:

Sam Keen: I wish I could begin by saying, "Damn you fear. Leave me alone!" But honesty demands that I address you as "Dear fear," for you have been with me most of my life. Now I want to understand

why I am attracted to you and did not banish you
long ago.

Fear: I am glad you are willing to admit that we are
reluctant friends. It has taken me some years to get
you to confess that you are a hesitant lover of what
you pretend to despise. What a capacity for self-
deceit you have, pretending that I was somehow your
fated enemy! Or, to be specific, that I was an unconscious legacy from your parents. Such transpar-
ent nonsense. If I am your fate, I am at least a fate
you have chosen and nurtured. It is not without your
consent and satisfaction that we have been together
all these years. You might have lived in conversation
with love, or courage, or creativity, or desire, or
fame. No! You have kept me around. So don't try
to disown me.

Sometimes we get into an anxiety rut by failing to play.
Our society teaches that work is good and, for adults, play
is evil. It is a sinful waste of time and talent. As we become
adults, we are supposed to grow out of our need for play.
If we don't, we are stupid and immature. The ultimate
believer in this has been called a workaholic. A workaholic
is a person who is not happy if he is not working at something. Such a person can't get enough of it to be satisfied.
This person may work long hours at one, two, or more jobs.
When he goes home, work from the office is taken along
and he thinks of things to do around the house. Idle time
makes a workaholic nervous. Weekends are an agony and
vacations drag because he can't wait to get back to work.
Housewives often show the same pattern, in working from
early morning until late at night seven days a week. They
attend to their houses and families excessively. No time is
left for resting. Workaholics have many of the same prob-

lems as alcoholics. Their obsession with work destroys their family and interpersonal lives, ruins their health (heart attacks, ulcers, and so on), and eventually leaves them desolate. In many cases, such a person would actually have been more productive *in the long run* if he didn't overdo working early in life.

As people have often pointed out, the word *recreation* means re-creation. The respite and escape we derive from play refreshes us and makes us able to go back and do more later. It enables us to be more productive longer.

It is interesting that a very common symptom of emotional disturbance is withdrawal. The person who is emotionally disturbed often isolates himself from friends, reneges on responsibilities, and turns off life. Such a person becomes unresponsive, uncommunicative, and unproductive. What has happened at this point is that problems have overwhelmed the person and he is unable to handle them. Thus, the person retreats from them and gives up completely. As is the case with many of the symptoms of emotional disturbance, this massive retreat from life is just an exaggeration of a more normal response that everyone has. We all need to get away from our problems and responsibilities from time to time. Play and recreation can be a "tactical retreat," enabling us to come back better and stronger later. If we use recreation that way, massive retreat into emotional disturbance will not be necessary. Thus, to live a productive life and keep anxiety at a minimum, we need to have adequate recreation and escape.

There are many ways we can do this. First, we need to relearn the way to play. If we have been anxious for a long time or are veteran workaholics, we may have to reach back into the past and search our memories to find things we can do for play. If we really think about it, we can come up with some. It is important that we begin to do things we like to do and that give us pleasure. Often they are things we have always wanted to do but couldn't seem to find time for.

Some people enjoy walks or hikes. Others like to play a sport such as tennis or golf. Some people like to go on picnics, while others would rather try out a new restaurant. Some people go to plays or movies for escape. Others prefer athletic events. Some take one- or two-day trips out of town, others prefer to stay home and play a family game or watch TV. Many people like to shop or browse. Some like to cook. Others like to listen to music or play an instrument. There are hundreds of things people do for recreation. You should do some of the ones you like. If it has been so long since you did them that you really don't feel like it, *force yourself.* You have to start somewhere.

When you engage in these activities, practice clearing your mind of all that has been preoccupying you. Then become totally absorbed in the activity you have chosen. It takes a little effort and practice to be able to do that, but you can train yourself to do so. Thought stopping, mentioned in chapter seven, is often helpful in keeping your mind clear of thoughts that would prevent you from enjoying play.

Once you learn to put worries out of your mind and become absorbed in play, you will find that these activities provide great satisfaction and enjoyment. They will add a new dimension of richness to your life. You will begin to see them as islands of refuge and refreshment. If you do them frequently, they become a major source of pleasure. You will be continuously thinking of the fun of the last experience and looking forward to the next. This makes life more exciting and enables us to do a better job at the more difficult tasks we face.

Developing a hobby can serve much the same purpose.

Many people find satisfaction, reward, fulfillment, and escape in a hobby. A survey done at the Menninger Clinic some years ago indicated that there was a positive relationship between being significantly involved in a hobby and good mental health.

It is also a good idea to participate in a wide variety of recreational activities. When children learn to play, they play alone at first. Later they develop parallel play; that is, they play at things alone but side by side. For example, they may each be swinging, playing with toy cars, or building sand castles, but they are not interacting with one another as part of the play. Still later, children begin to play together. They cooperate and interact in their play. As adults, we can use all of these types of play. We may want to have a hobby or some form of recreation that we do alone. In addition, we may want to read or paint or pursue some similar activity while family members or friends do something parallel. At other times, we will want to interact and cooperate, as in playing cards, chess, and so on. This satisfies our need for a variety of experiences in life. As we begin to have more fun, we will find that we are more relaxed and less anxious. Periodic escape from everyday problems refreshes us and allows us to see the problems of living in perspective.

Many people are so indoctrinated in the work ethic that they are not able to play or relax until they have first finished all their work. Of course, this is a trap because we never finish all our work. Consequently, we never have occasion to play. A good way to handle this is to develop work-play contingencies. To do this, you need to specify a given task or portion of a task that needs to be done. You then say to yourself, "When I finish that I will be entitled to a few hours of play for recreation and refreshment." You can then do the job and go play golf, go to a movie, or whatever you wish. Making play contingent on completing the work is good for a couple of reasons. First, it motivates you to get the work done quicker, and you are happier while you are doing it because you know that you are getting closer and closer to your recreation time. Second, you can enjoy the play without feeling guilty, because it is a reward for having done a significant job, which is now completed. Putting work and play in this type of juxtaposition makes for a productive and happy life-style.

Of course, you should also practice self-reinforcement at these times. Say to yourself, "That's good. I got the job done. I'm glad I did it. Now I'm going to go play golf. I'll get to that other job first thing tomorrow when I'm fresh and relaxed. It will go better then."

Be sure you don't set your goals too high. Some people pick a job that is too big to accomplish and still have enough time left over for play. The result, of course, is that they never quite get around to playing. If that is your problem, schedule a certain number of play hours after a specified number of hours of work rather than after completion of the job. You can say, "I'm going to work on the yard for four hours in the morning on Saturday. Then, I'm going to relax and watch the ball game on TV. What I don't get done in that four hours, I'll do next Saturday. But I'm really going to work hard during those four hours." If you do this, you will find that Parkinson's Law (work will expand or contract to fill the time provided to do it) often applies to this type of situation. If you have three or four things to do in the yard and have set no time limit, they may take all day. But if you set a four-hour time limit, you will generally get all or most of the work done in that amount of time, if you really try. Then you will have four hours for relaxation, and you've still accomplished the same amount in terms of work.

One final word: If you are determined to have fun in life, often you can approach work playfully and enjoy it more than you otherwise might. Suppose you have a rather boring task to do—perhaps peeling apples for a pie. If there are two people working at it, they can each take an equal number of apples and race to see who finishes first. The loser has to peel the remaining apples or clean up the mess afterward. This is, of course, a very simple example, but the point is that if you make an effort and use a little creativity, a lot of things in life can be approached playfully and enjoyed rather than endured. Such an approach to work and play is an antidote to much of the anxiety we experience daily.

12

Friends and Communication

HUMAN beings find considerable support and comfort in close relationships with others. The poet John Donne put it so well that his words have been quoted over and over:

No man is an island, entire of itself; every man is a piece of the continent, a part of the main; if a clod be washed away by the sea, Europe is the less, as well as if a promontory were, as well as if a manor of thy friends or of thine own were; any man's death diminishes me, because I am involved in mankind; and therefore never send to know for whom the bell tolls; it tolls for thee.

Having friends and being able to communicate meaningfully with them is a great bulwark against anxiety. It used to be that the immediate family and the extended family (aunts, uncles, grandparents, cousins, etc.) gave stability to people's lives and offered support in times of crisis. The extended family gave the individual a context in which to view himself or herself. There were frequent family gatherings, with stories about the history of the family and what various relatives had done and were doing. There was security in knowing that one was not alone. There were people who cared and who could be called upon for help in times of crisis such as births, deaths, illnesses, and financial problems. There were no questions asked. It was family. People did what had to be done to see one another through.

More recently, however, with the increased mobility of people the increasing tempo of our lives, and the breakdown of the nuclear family, the family is no longer able to fulfill such needs. Family members are scattered all over the country. They are busy with their own lives, and distance prevents them from developing a feeling of being closely tied to the others. The expense and disruption involved in coming to the aid of a cousin or a brother often seems too great a sacrifice. Many young people purposely arrange their lives so that they can be away from their families and on their own. As someone has said, Fate provides us with family; fortunately we can choose our associates. Yet facing crises without family can be very stressful and anxiety provoking.

For many people, friends take the place of the extended family. There are, of course, different levels of friendship. We all have a fairly large number of friends who are people we know in the sense that we recognize one another and carry on conversations when we happen to meet. There are other friends whom we enjoy being around sufficiently that we seek out occasions when we can meet. There are still other friends to whom we feel very close, with whom we share important aspects of our lives, and on whom we can call anytime we are in need.

Unfortunately many people have trouble making friends. There are, however, some rules that help in making and keeping friends. First, as is often pointed out, the best way to have a friend is to be a friend. That's an interesting turn of phrase, but it is important to understand what it means. It means that if we want to have friends, we need to do the things that make friends of people. When we meet people, we need to come out of our shell and become interested in *them* and their world. Often we are so preoccupied with our world and so concerned about whether we will make a good impression that we never really make contact with an individual we have just met. It is important to forget ourselves and reach out to others when we meet them. Try to find out who they are and what they are interested in. Remember, a stranger is just a friend you haven't met yet. Once we find out a little about someone, we can share some of our thoughts and experiences with that person. It also helps to smile a little and express pleasure about something the person mentions.

A second rule is that to develop friendships, we must develop a great deal of acceptance and patience. We must accept people as they are and not expect them to try to change to suit us. Fritz Perls put it very well when he said of others that they were not here to measure up to his expectations, nor he to theirs. He goes on to say that we are to do our own thing and be ourselves. If we develop a relationship in the process, that is wonderful; if not, it cannot be helped.

Of course, as a person gets to know and associate with us, she may change, but that must not be one of the conditions of friendship. Good friendship develops out of a certain amount of unconditional positive regard. When people do what we don't like, we could take offense, but it is necessary to overlook some things and forget them. We have to realize that people are "that way." They are not perfect. Because we are not perfect either, they also will have to overlook our shortcomings. We have to realize that people have faults and decide to be their friend anyway.

As friendship develops, you can strengthen and enhance it by doing small favors and showing little kindnesses to the person. Being able to accept similar favors from others graciously is the other side of the coin. Some people are quite willing to do things for others but cannot bring them-selves to let anyone do something for them. It is important to develop the ability to give and to receive.

Given the above rules for making friends, there are two further points to keep in mind. One is that to make friends we have to come in contact with people who are potential friends. We can't sit at home and expect them to come and find us. There are numerous ways to come in contact with potential friends. We can invite people to our home for dinner, parties, or get-togethers. We can go to places where we will meet people: Churches are good places, as are civic clubs, hobby groups, and discussion groups. If we get in-volved in community and social activities, we will make friends of some of the people we come in contact with.

The second point is that it is seldom possible to force friendship on someone. Friendship is a lot like a love re-lationship in this sense. Some people will like us, and a friendship will develop. Others, for a variety of reasons, will not, and a friendship will not develop. Real friendship has to be something that clicks between people. It cannot be forced and doesn't work if it is one-sided. We need to spend our time and energy selecting and developing friends from those who are interested, rather than lamenting the fact that some people we would like to be friendly with do not seem interested.

Psychologists frequently refer to friendship as being based on patterns of mutual reinforcement. Essentially this means that if the way a person looks, acts, thinks, and feels is pleasing to us, we will want to spend more time in that person's company. We say that being with this individual is fun. It is reinforcing and rewarding to us. If that person feels the same way about us, a friendship develops. This principle explains a lot of things about friendship. For ex-ample, our friendships change over the years. We may no longer enjoy being with people we once liked. People we once had little time for may come to be our best and closest friends. If we analyze what has happened, we may find that our interests, needs, and style of living have changed over the years, so that the type of person whose behavior is rewarding to us has changed. The principle of mutual reinforcement also explains why close friends can become bitter enemies (the line between love and hate is very thin). If our association with a person leads to mutual reinforcement, we become friends. If this person begins to thwart us in achieving or enjoying some important reward, however, we can become just as angry with the person as we were friendly before.

One of the best features of having friends is communication. Humans are the only animals that communicate by means of highly complex language and symbol systems. Hours spent in conversation with close friends are stimulating, rewarding, and anxiety reducing. Getting something off our chest by telling a friend about it makes us feel much better. Frequently friends are able to extend support or share some of their experiences with us. This can make a difference. Many times simply putting our thoughts into words clarifies our thinking and cuts through the nebulous quality of what is troubling us. When we clarify our thoughts and feelings, often they are seen to be not really so frightening. They seemed worse than they really were, mainly because we had not pinned them down and looked at them objectively.

Good communication between friends demands trust between the two. We need to feel free to tell our friends what we want to say. We need to be able to trust the friend to handle the information we give. Some people will be ruled out of this depth of friendship, but those we include will be people of special importance. Actually, a tragedy of many people's lives is that they often overlook the fact that a husband or a wife can be their best friend. That person is, after all, one who cares and is deeply involved with you for better or for worse. We may need to communicate with and cultivate our partner as one of our best friends. Strange to say, most marriage relationships unfortunately exist on a more superficial and defensive level than this.

While we need to have trust in our friends, they need to have empathy for us. Empathy is the ability to understand and fully appreciate how a person feels while still remaining objective about it. It is different from sympathy. In sympathy one feels the same emotion as the other person and becomes involved in the same experience as the other. This reduces the ability to be objective and to help the person effectively. For example, if someone is grieving and you sympathize with the person, you begin to grieve also. At that point, you both feel badly, and you are not able to help much. But if you were feeling empathy, you would fully appreciate how the person really felt but maintain enough objectivity to perceive the situation accurately. You would then be able to see workable solutions and go about putting them into operation. The result of empathy is help.

Communication involves two processes: talking and listening. People may have trouble with either or both. Some people have trouble talking. They find it difficult to put their ideas and feelings into words. Many times they don't know the right words to use. Other times they know the words but are afraid to say them for fear they will get an unfavorable response. If you have trouble talking, you need first to find a friend you trust and who has the ability to empathize with you. Then force yourself to talk to that person about your thoughts and feelings. You may start out with little things and short conversations, if you wish, and build up to more important and more extensive conversations later.

But you *must* begin to talk. Not even friends can read your mind.

Some people who find it difficult to talk, write letters and notes to others when an occasion arises. Often they can express their deeper feelings much more accurately this way. It is easy to do this by writing a note on a birthday, Christmas, or anniversary card. There are also cards designed just to say thanks or to send a brief thought to a person. In addition, you can write to others when you are out of town or they are, or during vacations, for example. A friend used to write notes to her husband and put them in with his lunch. He really looked forward to reading her notes while he ate. It gave both him and her a great lift each day.

The other side of communication is listening. We need to learn to listen to what people say to us. Sometimes this means just being quiet long enough for them to say what they want to. Often we have a tendency to interrupt or to jump to conclusions before the other person has finished talking. It is an art worth developing to be able to hear people out and let them say, in their own words, what they want to say. Of course, you also need to be sure that you really understand what they mean. Take in and carefully analyze what they are saying. Try to forget your own preconceptions and see things through their eyes and their value system so that you can really understand. It does no good to apply your own value system to the situation and discard as unimportant facts or details that the other person considers very important.

When you are not sure just how a person thinks or feels about something, try saying something like, "I'm not sure I follow, but what you seem to be saying is this. . . ." Then repeat the sense of what the other person said, as best you can interpret it. This technique gives the other person the opportunity to agree with or correct your statement.

Sometimes it is important to go behind the words another person is saying and tune in to the real underlying feelings. The tone of voice, physical posture, and gestures may all reveal anxiety, frustration, anger, joy, and other emotions that are not obvious from the words being used in the conversation. Generally if you pay attention to these cues you will communicate and understand much better. If you are pretty sure of the message coming from these cues, you can respond to the content of the words and the subtle cues without necessarily labeling them and making a major point of letting the person know you have picked them up. This often results in a feeling of warmth and friendship that says, "You understand me. I know you do. Thanks." Of course, you have to be sure you have correctly interpreted these cues, or you may eventually run into a blank wall or lose contact with the person. If you seem to be headed in that direction, it is often helpful to stop and say something like, "I'm not sure I fully understand. Do you seem to feel this way?" You can then label the feeling you think you picked up from the cues. The other person, again, can agree with or correct your impression.

In all relationships, it is possible for conflict or disagreement to develop. These situations can produce anxiety. One good way to resolve conflict is for the two people to stop before a bitter argument develops and do an exercise in which they take the role of the other person. Thus, with a married couple, the husband would argue his wife's side of the issue as persuasively as possible, as though he were her attorney or representative. His case for her side should include her feelings, views, arguments, reasons, and so forth. He should go beyond what she has actually said and add to her side. Following this, she should respond with clarification on points where he may have been inaccurate. She would then present his side of the issue, and he would provide clarification. This exercise almost always reduces the anger and promotes communication. The next step is to brainstorm (see chapter 9) for workable solutions.

Relationships based on positive regard, patience, trust, empathy, and effective conflict resolution are true and lasting friendships that comfort us in times of crisis and serve as bulwarks against many of the stresses of life.

Dr. Carl Rogers, a clinical psychologist, has studied and written extensively about such relationships. Many of his books are very helpful, especially *On Becoming a Person, Person to Person*, and *Becoming Partners: Marriage and Its Alternatives*.

13

Self-Hypnosis

★

HYPNOSIS is a very controversial area. Over the years the popularity of hypnosis in psychological treatment has waxed and waned. It has, from time to time, received wide attention and endorsement as a legitimate and useful therapeutic tool, only to fall into disrepute and disuse with the next generation of psychotherapists. There is currently considerable interest in hypnosis as a tool of treatment. Research is now going on in many important research centers that will enable us to understand the phenomenon better and use it effectively in therapy.

There are two main reasons why hypnosis frequently falls out of favor with therapists. One is that it has often been offered as a panacea for all kinds of problems. When it becomes apparent, after some scrutiny, that hypnosis is not a cure-all, many therapists seem to lose interest. The second reason is that we have never really established just what hypnosis is. Lacking a fully adequate understanding of its nature, many psychologists are reluctant to use it.

Some assert that hypnosis is an altered state of consciousness. They claim that a hypnotized person is in a trance, which gives the entranced person the ability to draw on the subconscious, or to alter brain chemistry and functioning. At the other extreme are people who say there is no such thing as hypnosis. They say the subject is just role-playing and responding to the suggestions of the hypnotist. These people have conducted research in the area and have been able to demonstrate that they can get their research subjects to do most, if not all, of the things hypnotized subjects do, but without ever hypnotizing the research subjects. Their subjects simply try very hard and are as cooperative as possible.

Before we present an overview of what hypnosis is, it is important to be clear about what it is not. There is hardly an area of psychology that is riddled with as many misconceptions as hypnosis.

First, hypnosis is not a form of sleep. Extensive studies of body reactions of the waking, hypnotic, and sleep states have demonstrated that hypnosis is not sleep, even though hypnotists often use the phrase "You are going to sleep" as part of the hypnotic-induction procedure. Hypnosis is closer to a waking state than to sleep, but it is not identical with being awake either.

Second, the experience of hypnosis is generally not a weird, mysterious, other worldly experience. Many stage hypnotists who perform primarily for entertainment play up this notion and encourage subjects to feel that way. This is not an intrinsic part of the process, however, and it seldom occurs when hypnosis is used in psychotherapy. It is a very normal, interesting, but unspectacular experience for most people. In fact, many times when I use it with patients, they require reassurance afterward that they were really hypnotized before they will believe it. It did not have the supernatural quality that they had always thought it would. By conducting certain tests of their reactions during the process, however, it is possible to verify that they were indeed hypnotized.

Third, a person who is hypnotized is not under the power of the hypnotist. The hypnotized person does not surrender his will or lose control of his own behavior. The person does become more susceptible to suggestion but basically only to the extent that he wishes to. If the hypnotist suggests that the person do something to which there are no strong objections, the entranced probably will do it. But if the hypnotist suggests something that the person really doesn't want to do, he simply won't do it. People are sometimes concerned that a hypnotist will take advantage of a person and get the person to do something antisocial or criminal. This is not possible if the person really doesn't want to do it. It is possible, however, to get people to do such things *with or without hypnosis* if they want to or can be persuaded to. Hypnotism has not been found to increase persuasibility toward this kind of behavior very much, if at all. Of course, a responsible hypnotist would not even suggest such a thing in any case. Thus, reports of hypnotism being used to involve people in crime or sexual activity are greatly exaggerated. Hypnotism isn't that powerful. As a precaution, however, against even the possibility, it is wise to deal only with a fully trained and responsible hypnotist such as a clinical psychologist, psychiatrist, or some other professional person.

Many people who think hypnotism has very special power are disappointed when they ask me to hypnotize them and tell them that they won't smoke anymore, drink anymore, or eat so much. It simply doesn't work that way.

Another frequent misconception is that a person will not remember anything about what went on during hypnosis after waking up. Actually, when the session is over the hypnotized person generally remembers everything that went on during the session. The only time one doesn't is when specific instructions are given by the hypnotist to not remember. This is referred to as posthypnotic amnesia. It occurs only when instructions to that effect are given or when the person firmly believes that that will be the effect. Even when the hypnotist gives instructions for posthypnotic amnesia, they don't always work. If you want to remember, you generally do. Posthypnotic amnesia is usually not called for in hypnotherapy but can be very useful on occasion. Often if I am working with a patient on an area that is very upsetting, I will induce posthypnotic amnesia for a period of time during the treatment until we get some of the problems resolved and they are not so painful to think about. This makes the patient more comfortable between sessions. In all other cases, they remember everything, and this is best because it facilitates the treatment.

Some people worry that if they become hypnotized they may not be able to wake up. Actually, this never happens. Some people who are hypnotized resist waking up at the end, often because they have found relief and escape in the hypnotic state and don't want to return to real life with its problems. This is quite rare, however. When it happens, the hypnotist can continue to work on bringing the patient out of it for a time. If that doesn't work, it is best to put the person in a comfortable place and wait. Generally he will fall asleep and later wake up alert. Or the person may rest in the hypnotic state for a while and then voluntarily come out of it. Nobody has gone into a hypnotic state and never come out.

People often say they have tried but can't be hypnotized. Some scientific literature claims a certain percentage of people cannot be hypnotized. It depends a lot on how one defines hypnosis. There are levels of hypnosis. Probably everyone, with the possible exception of some severely retarded or greatly emotionally disturbed individuals, can achieve some degree of hypnosis, even if it is very slight.

All right. How can we define hypnosis? First, we have to keep in mind that there is no adequate and perfectly clear definition. We simply don't understand the process well enough to define or explain it fully. But as a working definition for our purposes, it is useful to think of it as a heightened state of concentration accompanied by an increased ability to act on ideas and suggestions.

It is possible to think of a distraction-concentration continuum. At the extreme distraction end of the continuum people are very inefficient at performing even the simplest tasks. For example, if we had to walk across a stage, pour a glass of water, and give our name and address in front of an audience of 10,000 people, we probably would have great difficulty doing these very simple tasks because of the distraction and anxiety from the audience observing us. We might stumble across the stage (having forgotten how to walk), pour water on our wrist, throw the glass over our shoulder, and draw a blank on our name and address. At the other end of the continuum, when we are in deep concentration, we become very efficient and can accomplish tasks that are extremely challenging. Our complete concentration and the fact that we are engrossed in the task make it easy for us. Some people are able to get into this state of concentration easily. When they read a book or think about a problem, they shut out all extraneous stimuli from the environment. If you walk into the room and say something to them, they may not even hear you until you go over and shake them. These people are fast readers, good students, and good problem solvers. Other people, of course, are more easily distracted and less efficient in such tasks.

Examples of concentration are plentiful in athletes, also. For example, we often talk about a good baseball player being "off at the crack of the bat." When I played baseball, I was able to do that and found that I could reach fly balls that nobody expected me to. I did it by concentrating on the ball while it was still in the pitcher's glove. I then followed it with deep concentration through the wind up and during its path to the plate. When the ball was hit, I was off at once. In actuality, I was in a type of hypnotic state. Basketball players who stare at the basket, bounce the ball a couple of times, and take a few deep breaths are getting into a similar state before they shoot a foul shot. When they get into that state, crowd noise and attempted distractions do not bother them. They are able to go ahead and make the shot. Pass receivers in football have to have the same ability. If they try to run with the ball before they catch it, they usually drop it. Their concentration has been lost. We often say when they drop a pass that they heard the footsteps behind them—another example of disrupted concentration.

If we view hypnosis as a state of deep concentration on selected stimuli, it is easy to see why we can act more readily on suggestions and carry out ideas more efficiently under hypnosis. Viewing hypnosis in this way is a very useful working definition, whether it ultimately proves to be the final answer to the riddle of hypnosis or not. Hypnosis then becomes a way of inducing deeper concentration in ourselves at will, so that we can efficiently carry out tasks we want to.

There are thousands of ways to induce hypnosis. It is relatively easy for a skilled hypnotist to induce the state in a cooperative subject; it is also relatively easy for you to induce hypnosis in yourself.

One simple way to do this is to hold your hand at arm's length in front of your face at eye level. Then stare at a point on the hand. It can be any point such as a knuckle, ring, or freckle. The important thing is focusing vision on a spot. Then move the hand slowly toward your forehead and bring the point being focused on up to the forehead right between your eyes. When your hand touches your forehead, close your eyes, and go through the relaxation procedure outlined in chapter two. At this point you will be completely relaxed and your eyes will be closed. Now begin to count, and with each count let your body relax a little more and go a little deeper into the state of hypnosis. Beginners may want to count to forty-five or fifty. With a little practice you will be able to achieve satisfactory results by counting to only ten or fifteen. At the end of this procedure you will be in a light state of hypnosis. An alternate procedure is to roll the eyes back into the head as far as you can for a few seconds (rather than focusing on the hand and moving it to the forehead). Follow this with the same relaxation and counting procedure as above.

Once you achieve a light state of hypnosis, you can use it to relieve anxiety. One way is simply to tell yourself that you are going to calm down and get things under control. You will often find that this works wonders. When you wake up you will feel much better, less tense, and more relaxed.

You can also think through problems in this state and figure out ways to handle them. The relaxation and freedom from distraction will facilitate good problem solving.

In this state you can also tell yourself things that you know are true and would like to accept emotionally but have not been able to convince yourself of while awake. Hypnosis will make you more able to respond to such ideas or suggestions. For example, you might say to yourself, ''I'm going to interview for that job next week. There is no need to be overly anxious about it. It is normal to be a little tense in such a situation, and I'll be that. But I'll be more relaxed than I have in similar situations before. After all, the interview isn't that important. If I get the job, fine. If not, there is no sense in being anxious about it. Being calm will actually enhance my chances and make me more likely to handle the interview well and get the job. I'll be very calm. If I don't get it, maybe next time.'' Under hypnosis you can talk to yourself and tell yourself things of this sort. They will have a greater impact and be more believable. It's amazingly simple, but it works.

Some people also like to think about pleasant or calm situations and experiences under hypnosis. This is very similar to the meditation exercises discussed in chapter three. There is great similarity between hypnosis and meditation. In fact, many of the feats of the Yogis and other mystics are probably attributable to a type of hypnotic process.

After you have used hypnosis to help reduce your anxiety, it is simple to wake up. You simply say, ''I am now going to wake up. I will feel refreshed, relaxed, and wide awake. My mind will be clear, and I will feel good all over.'' Then open your eyes. You will feel as if you have just awakened from a nap or stopped working on something that completely engrossed your interest. It is a pleasant and exhilarating experience.

A word or two of caution is called for here: If hypnosis seems frightening to you or you are unsure of it, don't do it. It should be a pleasant, helpful experience. If it frightens you before you do it, or if it seems to have that effect when you try it, stop. Under such circumstances, it is best to consult a professionally trained hypnotist before going on. The professional may work with you and help you get over your fear, or the hypnotists may tell you that hypnosis is not for you at this time. If you have tried self-hypnosis and it didn't seem to work very well for you, it is also best to consult a professionally trained person. To find a qualified professional hypnotist, call the chairman of the psychology department at a nearby college or the head of the psychiatry department of a nearby medical school.

14

Professional Help

★

AFTER reading this book and trying some of the techniques that seem to fit your situation best, you may find that you are still experiencing more anxiety than you would like. You want to be calmer about things and relaxed enough to enjoy life rather than having it be such a struggle. Sometimes your anxiety may be related to a specific situation that will change after a short period of time. If that is the case, it may be best just to wait it out, much as you would a cold or some similar minor ailment. Everyone has short periods of stress and anxiety from time to time that have to be endured just as other unpleasant things in life must be. But if your anxiety is persistent, it may be best for you to seek help from a professional psychotherapist. Your problems may be such that they need more help than can be offered in a book like this. Or you may simply need a little help from someone with more experience in implementing the techniques outlined in this book. In any event, if you decide to seek professional help, there are some points worth considering.

The first place most people go with this type of problem is to their family physician or minister. While the family physician or minister can be very helpful, especially if the anxiety is relatively minor and not related to more serious problems, they may not be the best choice. The physician has had little or no training in psychotherapy but can often offer reassurance and advice based on the wisdom grown out of involvement with many people's lives. A physician can also prescribe medications that will reduce the discomfort you may be experiencing. These medications will be discussed in more detail later in this chapter. Some ministers are trained in counseling and can be very helpful; others do not have training or skills in these areas. The important thing to keep in mind is that the family physician and the minister are prepared to help with only minor, short-term anxiety problems, their major training and skills lie in other areas.

For people with more serious anxiety problems, the best source of help is generally a clinical psychologist, a psychiatrist, or a social worker. Numerous surveys have shown that most people are uncertain about what difference there is among these.

A clinical psychologist is a person who has earned a doctoral degree in psychology, with specialization in the areas of psychopathology, diagnostic evaluation, treatment of people with emotional disturbances, and related areas. This degree requires approximately ten years of academic training including thousands of hours of practical training and experience. The clinical psychologist must complete four years of undergraduate training in psychology and four or more years of graduate training in psychology. During the graduate training, in addition to relevant courses, the clinical psychologist works in treatment settings such as hospitals and clinics under the supervision of more experienced psychologists. She then completes a year of internship and undergoes an additional year or more of supervision after the doctoral degree is awarded. At this point, she can be licensed to offer services on an independent basis to the public. The clinical psychologist is trained and experienced in the basic sciences pertaining to diagnosis and treatment of emotional disturbances.

The psychiatrist is a physician who has decided to specialize in the treatment of people suffering from emotional disturbances. The psychiatrist, therefore, completes three or four years of undergraduate college, three- or four years of medical school, and generally a three or four-year psychiatry residency. As a resident the psychiatrist serves on the staff of a hospital or clinic and receives additional training and supervision in the treatment of emotional disturbances.

In terms of the rigor and extensiveness of their training, clinical psychologists and psychiatrists have essentially equivalent backgrounds. Both training programs are highly competitive, require a high degree of ability and diligence to complete, and take about the same number of years. The main difference is that one produces a psychologist who has decided to specialize in the treatment of emotionally disturbed individuals rather than one of the other areas of psychology, while the other produces a physician who has decided to specialize in the treatment of the emotionally disturbed rather than in one of the other areas of medicine. In most of their routine clinical practices, psychologists and psychiatrists function very similarly. But because their backgrounds are different, they do bring different skills to a situation. The physician is highly trained in the physical functioning of the body and is licensed to prescribe drugs. The psychologist is more highly trained in psychological functioning, personality theory, psychological diagnostic testing, and research. In many settings psychologists and psychiatrists work together in teams to capitalize on the unique skills of each. In independent private practice, they generally develop cooperative relationships to accomplish the same thing. For example, if a psychiatrist has a difficult diagnostic decision to make, she will frequently refer the patient to a psychologist for an extensive personality evaluation using psychological tests before the diagnosis is made. Likewise, if a patient of a psychologist has a physical problem or needs medication, the psychologist will have a physician see the patient and attend to this aspect. Both clinical psychologists and psychiatrists offer excellent help for the emotionally disturbed.

Social workers are also highly trained and very effective providers of mental-health care. To become a social worker one must complete four years of undergraduate training and two years of graduate training in social work. This leads to a Master of Social Work (MSW) degree. While it is possible to get a doctoral degree in social work the MSW is considered the terminal degree for clinical practice. The doctoral degree is more for research and academic social workers. During their graduate training, social workers receive extensive supervision in clinical work. To be licensed, they generally must be supervised for two years following completion of their MSW degree. A fully trained social worker should be licensed by the state to practice and be a member of the Academy of Certified Social Workers (ACSW). Social workers are trained to evaluate and treat emotional problems, including anxiety. Because their field has its roots in sociology, they often see cases where family therapy or marital counseling is required (psychologists and psychiatrists also see patients for this type of treatment).

Another type of practitioner that people often wonder about is the psychoanalyst. A psychoanalyst is a professionally trained person (usually a clinical psychologist or psychiatrist) who has had additional training and experience in the application of Freudian theory to the treatment of emotional disturbance. This usually involves two or three additional years of training and undergoing a personal psychoanalysis. Psychoanalysis generally requires several meetings a week for several years. Each session costs from $100 to $200, depending on the going rate in the area, the eminence of the therapist, and your ability to pay. Due to the time and expense involved in psychoanalysis, it is generally not indicated except for rather serious problems. In recent years the efficacy and efficiency of psychoanalytic treatment has come under serious question. Many psychologists and psychiatrists currently feel that the beneficial results are not sufficient to justify the time and expense required.

Another approach that is very useful in quelling anxiety is called behavior therapy. It has been developed primarily in the last twenty-five or thirty years and draws heavily on research from psychological laboratories throughout the world. Numerous investigations have demonstrated that behavioral treatments work effectively and in a relatively short period of time to bring relief from many types of emotional disturbance. Many of the ideas presented in this book are based on behavior therapy techniques.

Once you have decided to see a professional psychotherapist, the problem becomes one of choosing the person you want to see. They are, of course, listed in the yellow pages of the phone book, and friends can often recommend someone they know. You may also want to check with the local psychological, medical, or social work societies for names. There are also state psychological, medical, and social work associations. A little inquiry and some help from the telephone information operator will help you locate their offices. Another good way to look for a suitable professional psychotherapist is to write or call the chair of the psychology or social work department of a nearby college or university or the department of psychiatry at a nearby medical school. Tell them the general nature of your problem and the type of psychotherapist you would like to see. They are generally quite willing to help.

As noted earlier in this chapter, certain types of medication are used to reduce anxiety. Actually there are two major types of medication generally prescribed by physicians in such cases. These are sedatives and tranquilizers. Most sedatives are chemically benzodiazepines and have their effect by inhibiting and depressing the activity of the central nervous system (brain and spinal cord). They generally make a person feel calm. Some of the better-known brand names of these drugs are Librium, Valium, Serax, and Xanax. While technically these are sedatives are defined by their sedating effect on the central nervous system, they are often loosely referred to as tranquilizers or minor tranquilizers. Most of the real tranquilizers or major tranquilizers are chemically phenothiazine derivatives. Commonly known brand names of these are Thorazine, Mellaril, Stelazine, Trilafon, and Prolixin. How these drugs have their effect is not completely understood, but they seem to affect centers of the brain that are involved in expressing emotional behavior. When the emotion-mediating centers of the brain are better controlled, the person feels more tranquil and less confused. Buspar is a new medication that appears to be very effective in reducing anxiety but does not fit in either of the two major categories. Chemically it is quite different (technically an azaspiro-decane-dione).

One additional medication that your doctor may employ is called a beta blocker. Popular brands of this are Inderal and Tenormin. Chemically these are propranolol and atenolol hydrochlorides, respectively. They have their effect by blocking and reducing the effects of adrenaline on the autonomic nervous system. Adrenaline is what keys us up in threatening situations.

Usually sedatives, or minor tranquilizers and Buspar, are

used in cases of simple tension and anxiety. Major tranquilizers are used when the patient's agitation is accompanied by symptoms of thought disturbance, confusion, hostile or aggressive behavior, and other more serious forms of emotional disturbance such as psychosis. Beta blockers are better than the others for brief use in highly specific and infrequent stressful situations such as giving a major speech, getting married, taking an oral exam in graduate school, etc. It is best to trust your physician's judgment as to what is best for you at a given time.

Most people do not know that alcohol as found in the traditional alcoholic beverages of beer, wine, and whiskey is chemically a sedative drug. It has essentially the same effect as the drugs mentioned above, which are prescribed by a physician. As we are well aware, in our culture alcohol is a greatly abused and overused drug. The reason for this is that alcohol is a fast-acting, short-term sedative. Thus, the sedative effects of the drug occur very shortly after ingestion. But they also wear off before long. Therefore, to maintain the effect, we must drink more. The body habituates to such drugs. So before very long, larger and more frequent doses are required to get the same effect. At this rate you are apt to find yourself *addicted* to alcohol. It's a familiar pattern.

The important thing to keep in mind is that alcohol is a drug, specifically a sedative and one that we can become addicted to. Therefore, it is best not to use it as a self-medication. When we have anxieties and tensions, we should learn to handle them by using the techniques presented earlier in this book. If we need medication, we should see a physician. The physician can prescribe a safer medication that will work better. By using it under supervision, we can be assured that we are less likely to abuse the drug and become addicted. One should not take alcoholic beverages to relieve anxiety. That is too dangerous. If taken at all, alcoholic beverages are best in moderate amounts with meals or on social occasions for added pleasure, rather than as desperate attempts to escape from pain and anxiety.

Another very important point is that drugs frequently interact with one another when taken together. Many times two drugs that are quite safe and helpful if taken separately can become extremely potent and dangerous if taken together. Alcohol is very much this way with some of the sedatives and tranquilizers mentioned above. If one takes a small dose of some of these medications and then drinks a few ounces of alcohol, the combined effect can cause the person to be dangerously slow in reactions, making driving, working, or other activities very hazardous. A person may also lose consciousness and in some cases even die as a result. Be very careful about taking medications concurrently or with alcohol. Ask your physician before you do.

One other form of self-medication should be mentioned. There are various patented medicines on the market that are available in drugstores without a prescription. They are sold to relieve tension and to aid in going to sleep. Most of these contain small doses of antihistamines, which are known to produce a sedative effect. Many of them also contain other mild sedative agents, small amounts of pain-relieving medications, and sometimes vitamins. If you are experiencing very mild and temporary tension and anxiety, these are certainly worth a try. They may help to make stronger measures unnecessary. Your druggist can help you select one. They are reasonably safe and very economical. Be sure to use them as directed on the package. They should *be used only for brief periods of time*. If the problem persists more than a week or two, consult your physician.

The medications discussed above are primarily palliative rather than curative. That is, they will make you feel a little better temporarily, but they do not cure or clear up the problem. If the anxiety is brief and infrequent, they can be very helpful. But if it persists or comes back too often, chances are you need psychotherapeutic treatment by a clinical psychologist, psychiatrist, or social worker. The sooner you find one and begin to work on your problems, the sooner you will feel better. Psychotherapy for anxiety-related problems is essential because many of the medications can be addictive if used over long periods of time. When this occurs, the problems with the cure are worse than the disease.

One final point should be mentioned before we end this book. That is that many people who work very hard alone or with professional help at reducing anxiety often report that when the anxiety begins to go down, depression begins to increase. This occurs in only a small number of cases, and it should not be a matter of great concern. Usually what has happened is that the person has been so accustomed to living under great tension or pressure, that a normal anxiety-free state seems flat and drab. Then they get depressed. Generally if one is patient the depression will leave. It helps to involve yourself in things you enjoy and begin to make life more interesting and exciting. The points made in chapter eleven can be helpful. If the depression is unusually severe or persistent, you should contact a professional psychotherapist.

Be cool.

Index

About the Author

DR. C. EUGENE WALKER received his Ph.D. in Clinical Psychology from Purdue University in 1965. He is currently Professor of Psychology at the University of Oklahoma Medical School and Director of Pediatric Psychology there. In addition, he maintains a private and consulting practice of psychology. He has contributed numerous articles to professional journals in the field of psychology and has authored several books.

IMPORTANT BOOKS FOR TODAY'S WOMAN

___**THE FEMALE STRESS SYNDROME** by Georgia Witkin, Ph.D.
0-425-10295-5/$3.95
Do you suffer from headaches, PMS, crippling panic attacks or anxiety reactions? Dr. Witkin tells of the stresses unique to women, and why biology and conditioning may cause the strains of daily life to strike women twice as hard as men.

___**THE SOAP OPERA SYNDROME** by Joy Davidson, Ph.D.
0-425-12724-9/$4.95
The learned behavior of drama-seeking is the need to fill out lives with melodrama. Rid your life of unnecessary crises, end the heartache of addictive relationships, discover your own specialness and self-worth, strengthen intimacy with your partner...and much more.

___**BEYOND QUICK FIXES** by Georgia Witkin, Ph.D.
0-425-12608-0/$4.95
Is a dish of ice cream your answer to a frustrating day at work? Does buying new lipstick help you forget your overdrawn checkbook? Thousands of women rely on a "quick fix" to feel comforted or in control—instead of facing problems head-on. Find out how to change these temporary fixes into real, long-term solutions.

___**BEATING THE MARRIAGE ODDS** by Barbara Lovenheim
0-425-13185-8/$4.99
In this practical, clear-sighted book, the author offers a simple, down-to-earth plan for women who want to take charge and achieve their personal goals of marriage and family. The truth is, opportunities abound for women who know the real facts—and know how to use them.

___**SLAY YOUR OWN DRAGONS: HOW WOMEN CAN OVERCOME SELF-SABOTAGE IN LOVE AND WORK** by Nancy Good
0-425-12853-9/$4.99
For many women, love and success seem like impossible dreams. Leading psychotherapist Nancy Good shows that self-destructive behavior may be the unconscious cause. Now you can achieve happiness by unveiling the self-sabotage in love, career, health, emotions, money and compulsions.

For Visa, MasterCard and American Express orders ($15 minimum) call: 1-800-631-8571

FOR MAIL ORDERS: CHECK BOOK(S). FILL OUT COUPON. SEND TO:	**POSTAGE AND HANDLING:** $1.75 for one book, 75¢ for each additional. Do not exceed $5.50.
BERKLEY PUBLISHING GROUP 390 Murray Hill Pkwy., Dept. B East Rutherford, NJ 07073	**BOOK TOTAL** $ ____
NAME_____	**POSTAGE & HANDLING** $ ____
ADDRESS _____	**APPLICABLE SALES TAX** $ ____ (CA, NJ, NY, PA)
CITY_____	**TOTAL AMOUNT DUE** $ ____
STATE_____ZIP_____	**PAYABLE IN US FUNDS.** (No cash orders accepted.)
PLEASE ALLOW 6 WEEKS FOR DELIVERY. PRICES ARE SUBJECT TO CHANGE WITHOUT NOTICE.	388